Palliative
Care
Assessment:

*Spiritual Impact in the Lives of Patients
with Cancer at Roswell Park
Comprehensive Cancer Center*

Palliative Care Assessment:

*Spiritual Impact in the Lives of Patients
with Cancer at Roswell Park
Comprehensive Cancer Center*

RENINGER FLORES
AND PAUL SPITALE

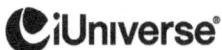

PALLIATIVE CARE ASSESSMENT: IMPACT IN THE LIFE OF PATIENTS WITH CANCER AT ROSWELL PARK COMPREHENSIVE CANCER CENTER

iUniverse books may be ordered through booksellers or by contacting:

iUniverse
1663 Liberty Drive
Bloomington, IN 47403
www.iuniverse.com
844-349-9409

ISBN: 978-1-6632-3745-3 (sc)
ISBN: 978-1-6632-3746-0 (e)

Library of Congress Control Number: 2022904974

Print information available on the last page.

iUniverse rev. date: 04/14/2025

CONTENTS

LIST OF TABLES

BIOGRAPHY

Dr. Paul R. Spitale II, Ph.D.

Dr. Paul Spitale served as the Life Recorded Program Coordinator at Roswell Park Comprehensive Cancer Center (a storytelling program geared toward recording and archiving the stories and lives of hospital staff, patients, and their families) from 2020 to 2024. He is an educator, counselor, business owner, consultant, speaker, actor, musician, DJ, father, and highly driven knowledge-seeker. For nearly two decades, Dr. Spitale has been an educator. He teaches college and high school writing and film courses. He was the Education Director at the nonprofit BEAM (Buffalo Engineering Awareness for Minorities) where he worked for over 13 years creating award-winning STEM courses for underrepresented students in the Western New York State area. His drive and passion for writing and storytelling stems from his life-long experience with creating poetry, music, screenplays, short stories, academic papers, films and award-winning documentaries. His work also earned him an Emmy Nomination for the documentary entitled "When I See You: A Cancer Patient's Journey" viewable on YouTube (youtube.com/watch ?v=OtDXVPUN6wE). Dr. Spitale states that "storytelling is a voyage that few dare to embark. Like many voyages, the journey itself is much more important than the destination. Watching one's story unfold in the moment is a powerful way to experience and understand what is occurring in the world."

PREFACE

My coauthor, Reverend Doctor Reninger Flores was born in Tarapoto, Peru. He began his studies at the Peruvian Union University where he received his Bachelor of Theology degree. He then earned a Master of Divinity Studies at the Adventist American Latino Seminary, headquartered in Brazil. Rev. Dr. Flores worked for eleven years as a District Pastor in the Northern Peruvian Conference of the Seventh-day Adventist and five years in the Adventist Development and Relief Agency of Peru (ADRA-PERU). He then graduated with a Master of Divinity degree with an emphasis in Applied Theology at Logos Christian University, in Orlando, Florida, USA. Finally, he earned his Doctor of Ministry degree at Andrews University in Berrien Springs, Michigan, USA. He currently works as a Chaplain at Roswell Park Comprehensive Cancer Center and is the creative founder of the Virtual Buffalo International Hispanic Church operated out of Buffalo, New York, USA. He is married to his loving wife Mary Esteves and together they raised four beautiful children: Elina, Hulda, Mary, and Daniella.

On the surface, author Rev. Dr. Reninger Flores or "Reni" as I know him, is a kind, caring, loving, selfless individual who goes out of his way for others. However, if you get the privilege to talk to him, to be in his presence, and to know him as a colleague and friend as I do, you see the complexity in his eyes, hear the strength in his voice, and feel the depth in his soul. Rev. Dr. Flores is a man who has experienced much in his life: joy, heartache, achievement, loss, happiness, and pain. He has endured the unthinkable, yet does not bear any negative scars this would leave on any one of us and (likely because) his faith is unwavering. His experiences have shaped him into the man we see before us and God shines through his tireless work. As a Chaplain at Roswell Park Comprehensive Cancer Center, Rev. Dr. Flores sees a lot of suffering and pain as well as joy and hope. The empathy he exudes for his patients comes from a place of faith, love and adversity.

When Dr. Flores first asked me to help in the editing of his English translation of the book, I was beyond delighted to lend any of my skills to him and to the telling of our story as colleagues. Our patients and colleagues hold Dr. Flores in the highest regard as he truly walks in the life and teachings of Christ. I am sincerely a better man for being able to call Rev. Dr. Flores my colleague, my coauthor, and more importantly, my friend.

Paul R. Spitale II, Ph.D.
Professor of Writing
State University of New York College at Jamestown

Palliative Care Assessment: Impact in the Life of Patients with Cancer at Roswell Park Comprehensive Cancer Center

ABSTRACT

PALLIATIVE CARE ASSESSMENT: SPIRITUAL IMPACT
IN THE LIVES OF PATIENTS WITH CANCER AT
ROSWELL PARK COMPREHENSIVE CANCER CENTER

by Reninger Flores and Paul Spitale

Advisor: Vaughan Grant

ABSTRACT OF GRADUATE STUDENT RESEARCH

Dissertation

Andrews University

Seventh-day Adventist Theological Seminary

Title:

PALLIATIVE CARE ASSESSMENT: SPIRITUAL IMPACT IN THE LIVES OF PATIENTS WITH CANCER AT ROSWELL PARK COMPREHENSIVE CANCER CENTER

Name of researcher: Reninger Flores

Name and degree of faculty adviser: Vaughan Grant, DMin Date completed: May 2020

Problem

This study investigated the understanding and use of spiritual care assessment in palliative care patients. Having a conscious and accurate palliative care assessment was always a big challenge in the chaplaincy community. It is the most visible and important part of the chaplaincy and as a result, the care we provide can become fruitful and spiritually powerful for the patient and for the network that supports the patient. It is the express desire that Roswell Park Comprehensive Cancer Center continue providing the best tool that will allow chaplains to perform their duties with honorable outcomes.

I reviewed the most important works about assessment in general; however, focusing on the area of palliative care, there were a few that were also reviewed and analyzed with the purpose of getting information that is particularly applicable at the Cancer Center.

Method

During 2018, a questionnaire with 34 questions was developed and distributed to six professional chaplains and 24 spiritual care volunteers who have close weekly interaction with palliative care patients. In addition, samples of the Palliative Care Patient Census Report were collected on a daily basis. The chaplains and volunteers had three to four months to return the questionnaires with the answers and personal observations. The participants were mainly cooperative and dedicated time to reading and answering the 34 questions divided into four sections: Environment, Sources of Support, Academic Training, and Preparation. Support was often conditional with common concerns related to informed consent—the protection of anonymity, and confidentiality; the right to withdraw from research; and ownership of the samples. I sent a Thank-You card to all the participants.

Results

In all, 27 participants returned the completed questionnaires in sealed envelopes. The participants were mainly cooperative and dedicated time to reading and answering the 34 questions. Among the volunteers who visited palliative care patients, there was an average of 11 years of experience, and 7 years of educational preparation. Only 57% had CPE studies and 43% had any kind of theological preparation such as an MDiv; there was one PhD in Religious Education. This research also showed that only 43% of the medical team clearly understood the role of the chaplains in the hospital, and 71% of the respondents agreed that human psychology is also very important when chaplains interact with patients during assessment and reassessment. Another interesting piece of information is that the average age in the cancer population at Roswell is 54 in females and 60 in males.

Conclusions

This study demonstrated that knowledge and understanding of spiritual care assessment in palliative care patients was limited in Roswell Park Comprehensive Cancer Center, but that there is, at present, a desire to continue to understand much better the importance of these assessments. I concluded that an improved palliative care assessment would contribute to better outcomes when assessing and following-up with patients, especially given that 42% of the population was Roman Catholic and 59% were non-Catholic. I suggest that more studies be developed in areas of palliative care assessment.

Andrews University

Seventh-day Adventist Theological Seminary

PALLIATIVE CARE ASSESSMENT: SPIRITUAL IMPACT
IN THE LIVES OF PATIENTS WITH CANCER AT
ROSWELL PARK COMPREHENSIVE CANCER CENTER

A Project Document Presented in Partial Fulfillment of
the Requirements for the Degree Doctor of Ministry

by Reninger Flores May 2020

PALLIATIVE CARE ASSESSMENT: SPIRITUAL IMPACT
IN THE LIFE OF PATIENTS WITH CANCER AT
ROSWELL PARK COMPREHENSIVE CANCER CENTER

A project document presented in partial fulfillment of
the requirements for the degree Doctor of Ministry

by Reninger Flores

APPROVAL BY THE COMMITTEE:

_____   _____

Adviser,   Director of DMin Program
Vaughan Grant   Hyveth Williams

_____   _____

Alanzo Smith   Dean, SDA Theological Seminary
                                 Jiří Moskala

                                 _____

                                 Date approved

DEDICATION

I want to dedicate this project to the memory of my daughter Elina Del Pilar Flores de Nina who is resting until Jesus comes back. She made me promise to finish it. I also dedicate it to Hulda Karina Guash, patient mother and example of resilience and faith; Mary Indira Insalaco, intellectual, counselor, and mother of two precious children; Ruth Daniella Harner, dedicated mother, entrepreneur, and expert in modern technology; to my wife Mary Esteves de Flores, exemplary mother and devoted Christian who patiently gave me the time I needed to finish this project; and also to my sons-in-love, Jason, Jorge, Alberto, and Luke, who have always been a great support during times of discouragement.

ACKNOWLEDGMENTS

The present finished project was made possible due to many people who dedicated time during my journey as a student at Andrews University. My first acknowledgement is to God, the one who gave me energy, hope, mission, and vision to accomplish this job. Dr. Mario Cevallos made it possible for me to enroll in the DMin program, Chaplaincy cohort at Andrews University. I also want to recognize Dr. Alanzo Smith, Executive Secretary of the Greater New York Conference, and Dr. Vaughan Grant, ACPE Associate Supervisor and adjunct professor at SDATS, the Florida Hospital Division Center for Pastoral Education. They were the two readers for my project and gave me many helpful observations and suggestions. I would also like to acknowledge the Roswell Park Comprehensive Cancer Center. Dr. Elizabeth Lenegan, Director of Spiritual Care Services, first opened the door for me to work as Staff Chaplain and also to carry out the Palliative Care Assessment Survey that I used in this project. Rev. Melody Rutherford, MDiv, chaplain at Roswell Park Cancer Institute, Rev. Joseph Blatz, MDiv, chaplain at South Mercy Hospital; Fr. Ray Corbin from the Infant of Prague Roman Catholic Church, Cheektowaga, New York, and Dr. Paul Spitale, Coordinator of Life Recorded Program at Roswell Park, never hesitated to give me their precious time and encouragement when I needed it. I also appreciate the great support of Leonard Caruana, CIM IRB Multisite Research Administrator, and the

Office of Research Subject Protection at Roswell Park, who played a big role in the approval of my research.

I would also like to offer special thanks to Sr. Judith A Terrameo OSF, MAPM, BCC, and chaplain at Mount St Mary's Hospital, Lewiston, New York, for her continued support in her desire to see me finish this project and receive my degree. I would also like to thank Dr. David Penno, my Andrews University advisor, for his oversight ad help. I am grateful. To my wife Mary Esteves who has waited patiently for me to finish this project after all the time-consuming hours, days, and obstacles that presented themselves as I worked on this project. Finally, I would like to thank Averil Kurtz and Camille Clayton for the work they did to finish he last part of this project.

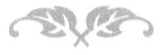

CHAPTER 1
INTRODUCTION

This is an idea of how I developed the proposal which includes resources used to create the format of the body content, the time, methods, and anything that helped to get results for this research. I consider that effort was very productive allowing me to understand much better what palliative care assessment means.

Description of the Ministry Context

Roswell Park Comprehensive Cancer Center treats and researches cancer anomalies. It was founded in 1889 by Dr. Roswell Park. The hospital is considered the only comprehensive cancer center in upstate New York. The Institute has 3,221 employees, including 308 faculty members and 306 nurses. Located in downtown Buffalo, New York, Roswell Park Comprehensive Cancer Center offers its services to a vast population of 259,384 residents, together with other patients coming from more than 40 states nationwide. The vast majority of residents are Caucasians, followed by African Americans, Hispanics, Asians, and Native Americans. Roswell has eight floors that include ICU, a post-operatory area, research for new trial treatments such as immunotherapy, and so on. Roswell also takes care of patients who are receiving chemotherapy treatments on a daily basis. They use the fourth and fifth floors in the building for this purpose. However, in order to reach the community, Roswell has a satellite site in Amherst. This is my fifth year working as a staff member in the Spiritual Care Department. I am also a member of the Patients Palliative Care and Disaster Mental Health teams. The rest of the staff includes the director of the Spiritual Care Department, a Roman Catholic priest, and a Pentecostal Church Reverend.

Statement of the Problem

Appropriate palliative care spiritual assessment is required at Roswell Park Comprehensive Cancer Center. For many years it was not a regular requirement for the work of the Spiritual Care Department until the Joint Commission on Accreditation of Healthcare Organizations (JCAHO) recommended it. The JCAHO wanted to see a practical spiritual assessment of palliative care patients in practice. According to the Roswell Park Comprehensive Cancer Center, most of the departments, including the Spiritual Care Department, have different assessments plans, and the results are positive.

Statement of the task

The task of this project was to develop, implement, and evaluate a palliative care spiritual assessment plan that could be used by chaplains, volunteers, and other members of the spiritual care team at the time of the initial visit with palliative care patients at Roswell Park Comprehensive Cancer Center.

Delimitations

The Palliative Care Spiritual Assessment Plan would be used for the Daily List (DL) of the new admittees as palliative care patients at Roswell Park Comprehensive Cancer Center. The plan was used without discrimination of gender, race, age, or economic status. The study was carried out over two years, starting in 2014.

Description of the Project Process

A. In order to prepare the palliative care spiritual assessment for the new patients in the palliative care unit, the following procedures were reviewed by the palliative care team.

B. A theological basis for the spiritual assessment was developed. This was examined in both scriptural and recent theological studies. The biblical basis was Matt 5:13, 48; 7:24-29; Mic 6:6; and E. G. White writings such as Counsels on Health and Steps to Christ.

C. Current literature was reviewed and included research on the theological and sociological basis for spiritual assessments and current spiritual assessment models such as the Faith, Influence, Community, and Address (FICA) model and the Holy Spirit Assessment. Psychological research regarding spiritual care in hospitals such as the Personal View Survey (PVS) was also carried out to assess hardiness and the Sense of Coherence Scale (SOC), and Seeking of Noetic Goals (SONG), and looking at the overall meaning in life. Additional analysis included ethical implications of a spiritual care assessment, using the Source of Meaning Profile (SMP), and the most applied trends in reference to spiritual care assessments.

D. A sheet summarizing the complete psychological, sociological, and spiritual profile with clearly defined areas of assessment of the patient and their family was developed. This included four aspects of each area of assessment: (a) demographics, (b) spiritual background of the patient, (c) current weak and strong areas of spirituality, and (d) ways to fulfill the spiritual needs of the patient.

E. Three spiritual care directors were interviewed to discover their knowledge about palliative care spiritual assessment. They included one from the hospital where I was working, another hospice director, and finally, another hospital director in the area. The primary purpose of this survey was to have an idea of how they were fulfilling the needs of the palliative care patient and how beneficial it was to have a unified spiritual care assessment. I sought to include directors of the most prominent hospitals in the Buffalo area, and my goal was to finish this section in December 2015. Writing the project document continued after this date, but the development, implementation, and evaluation phases were to be finished by then.

F. From the responses, conclusions were drawn concerning the expectations of the various site directors, as well as what the best way was to support the palliative care patients. From these conclusions, a model of spiritual care assessment for palliative care patients materialized. This model was customized according to the needs of Roswell Park Comprehensive Cancer Center as a spiritual care provider and the recommendations of the JCAHO.

G. The spiritual care assessment was implemented at Roswell Park Comprehensive Cancer Center for a period of one year.

H. The effectiveness of the spiritual care assessment for palliative care patients was evaluated at Roswell Park Comprehensive Cancer Center over a period of one year. Once a week, on Wednesdays, I had the opportunity to conduct assessments using the new survey created, and the data was stored in the files of the Pastoral Care Department. Once a year, the Roswell Park commission of evaluation, composed of the Hospital Director, the Palliative Care Director, the Psych-Oncologist Director, the Pastoral Care Director, and the staff chaplains, met to evaluate the project.

I. This project was completed in December 2015. 4

Definition of terms

We used the most common hospital terminology and provided the meanings for those who needed necessary clarification.

ICU: Intensive Care Unit

JCAHO: Joint commission on Accreditation of Health Care Organizations

ECMC: Erie County Medical Center

DSM: Diagnostic and Statistical Manual of Mental Disorder QOL: Quality of Life

RMP: Road Map Plan

WNY: Western New York

DNV: Do Not Visit

CAM: Complementary and Alternative Medicine

EOL: End of Life Patient

WHO: World Health Organizations

PC: Palliative Care

PPACA: Patient Protection and Affordable Care Act

R/S: Religious and Spiritual

HIPAA: Health Insurance Portability and Accountability Act

CHAPTER 2

THEOLOGICAL REFLECTION ON PALLIATIVE CARE ASSESSMENT

There are many instances where the Bible portrays the validity of the assessment activity, especially when a minister is trying to perform a responsible and competent intervention on behalf of a patient. Johns (2004) mentioned that "being mindful, easing suffering is an essential resource for professionals working with the seriously ill and the dying" (para. 1). Palliative care assessment is a vital tool in the process of creating an individualized patient plan. This is required from a medical standpoint, and I do not see any reason for patients not to have the same care when chaplains are doing their job and creating a follow-up plan for them. In the entire Bible, from Genesis to Revelation, God's agents and great prophets were engaged in these concerns, and God Himself is always assessing, planning, goal-directing, and following up. The same is seen at many mental health agencies that are dedicated to helping people who suffer from any kind of mental issues, physical disability difficult situations like being on the verge of becoming homeless. They have both goal-oriented interventions and drop-in centers.

In the first case, all the customers have to have a mental health diagnosis provided by any mental health agency (Lake Shore Rehabilitation, Horizon, ECMC, etc.) and goals that have to be evaluated every quarter/semester of the year with continuous customer progress notes. Basic courses in principles of psychosocial rehabilitation were indicated to be learned during the year. In the second case, drop-in centers (Harbor House, Heaven House, City Mission, etc.), goals are not necessary, but attention to the customer's present needs should also be monitored in a very careful way. There must still be an idea and record of the people they are serving, and earlier referrals are likely. In drop-in centers, progress notes are not usually required. Working with minds regarding spiritual concerns or discovering the underlying realities of assigned patient where multiple factors are involved is a very challenging process. For example, schools trying to assess bullying situations found that "the reality of assessing a complex, underground behavior involving multiple participants and influenced by multiple factors is that there not be no single 'gold standard' for accuracy" (Mayavu, 2017, p. 53). Mental health settings and research about diagnosis should be taken seriously when a patient's quality of life is in jeopardy.

In focus is the debate on mental health related to universalism and relativism concerning the nature and function culture plays in diagnosis, primarily through analysis of the changes in the mental health diagnostic system: the Diagnostic and Statistical Manual of Mental Disorders (DSM). Clinicians use the DSM to diagnose and classify mental health problems, mental disorders, and to plan treatment strategies. (DeMarinis, 2018, para. 1).

However, in the chaplaincy arena, there are not many options to check. Chaplains need to have a plan, and the plan of intervention will come with previous assessment (the admission interview), as well as every two weeks or whenever it is necessary to make a re-assessment. Because of their need to preach a sermon every weekend, pastors never do so without previous rigid preparation and assessment of their audience if they are conscious of their calling.

Perhaps there might be the possibility of extenuating circumstances that could change the trajectory of the sermon.

Some of the benefits of planning your sermonic year are being able to avoid the rush and panic that comes with not knowing what you will be preaching about next week. This also allows time for the worship and communication coordinators to plan services and branding that will contribute to the theme. Finally it allows for a balance in the topics and spiritual lessons presented. (Kidder, 2015, p. 22)

If there is not a previous assessment and a traced plan in either mundane affairs or holy endeavors, the results can be seriously minimized or jeopardized and can produce disappointments for both parties (chaplain and patient). Some of the currents assessments are also more monoculturalistic than multiculturalist in approach, as mentioned by Gaithri (2012): "The current GMH research agenda appears to be using a monocultural model that is individualistic, illness-oriented, and focused on intrapsychic processes. Ironically, issues of culture are prominently absent in many discussions of global mental health" (para. 1). Think about God's creating this world, but also addressing the possibility of chaos with the entrance of sin as a result of disobedience deliberately promoted by Satan. The Trinity made the plan of creation and assessed the situation of sin, but the Bible clearly declares that Jesus came to this world to save humanity. However, this plan was not a Code Blue Call or 911 emergency call; it was formulated during the eternal deliberations. "According as he hath chosen us in him before the foundation of the world, that we should be holy and without blame before him in love" (Eph 1:4).

Still, the plan of redemption where the Son of God was appointed to come to this world and to die in our favor was not a last-minute plan. It was a deliberate assessment of the situation, a goal-oriented activity that involved a "determinate counsel and foreknowledge of God" (Acts 2:23; Gal 4:4) before anything happened. God is a God of prevention. We have a God of planning, goal-oriented, with follow-up endeavors, and so on. Everything in His schedule included the end of this world that only the Father knows.

As people who belong to God, we always have to understand that our entire life span is in God's hands. There are cases in hospitals from time to time where the family wants to prolong the life-suffering of patients after the doctors have said there is nothing more that can be done.

For those people, who, by faith, believe in either an impersonal higher power, cosmic force, or ultimate concern, or a personal Transcendent other, or God, this transcendent domain of SWB embraces the other three and provides depth of understanding and wellbeing. (Stark & Bonner, 2010, pp. 265-277)

When God decides to heal you, He will use simple or complicated things to perform His will, but when the time is over, the time to sleep has arrived (John 11:11), no one and nothing can stop it. No one can guarantee a patient's healing because the entire church is praying for the patient. We need to ask for the will of God. His sovereignty takes precedence over any human endeavor. Some lives will be healed for the glory of God; others will wait for the eternal resurrection when "the Lord Himself shall descend from heaven, with the shout, with the voice of archangel, and with the trump of God: and the death of Christ shall rise first" (1 Thess 4:16).

Western philosophy portrays a birthday as a cause of joy and praise, but the time of death as a time of desperation and sadness has no biblical support. However, we all agree that "sharing memory is what it means to love" (Glickman, 2012, p. 2). What a magnificent blessing! Both are sacred moments and need to be respected and enjoyed. That was reason enough for the Psalmist to declare: "So teach us to number our days, that we may apply our hearts unto wisdom" (Ps 90:12). God planned when every human being would appear in this world, but also when he or she has to depart. Our time to accomplish our duties is time-framed, programmed, and evaluated.

Perhaps the most famous story associated with these discussions relates the time when Rabbi Judah Ha-Nasi lay dying. His disciples gathered at the gates of his home to pray for him. The Rabbi's maidservant, seeing that the tumult was actually interfering with the natural process of life's ending, may her way to the roof of the house. Once there, she took hold of a large clay pot and threw it with all her might off the roof. It crashed upon the ground. The disciples, startled by the noise, stopped their prayers. At the moment, Rabbi Judah's soul departed. From this we learn that there comes a time where is appropriate to allow the flame of life to flicker out. There is as Ecclesiastes reminds us, "a time to be born and a time to die." (Simcha, 2019, p. 273)

The entire Bible is full of amazing inspirations. Daniel and Revelation are full of detailed symbolism and numerology that indicate nothing was done in chaos; everything was planned, systematic, and goal-oriented. Daniel 2 is a vivid example of how God works with the history of humankind. Nothing is left to accidental endeavor. It is planned, assessed, and accomplished. Six hundred years before the Lord was born in Bethlehem of Ephrata, the prophecies declared every step of the Savior in detail (Mic 5:2). According to God's schedule, human history had to follow the blue print found in Daniel (Dan 2). First came the downfall of the Babylonian Empire (605-538 BCE), then the fall of the powerful Medo-Persian kingdom (538-476 BCE); the next empire in the plan was the violent Greco- Macedonian conquerors (476-176 BCE). The last earthly empire that was prophesied was the Roman Empire (476 BC- 538 CE) that was divided into ten other small kingdoms that formed part of modern Europeans countries. God is not a God of improvisations. He is a God of order, planning, and follow-up. The same is seen in Dan 4 and best, in Dan 8:14. God's plan seems well organized and meticulously planned.

October 22, 2029 will mark 176 years that the Seventh-day Adventist Church has been preaching to the world that Jesus is coming again. Many believers think that Jesus' coming has delayed too long; others are leaving the church and many act like their faith is fading. I embraced this message in 1974, and it was confirmed with a dream of Jesus' coming to this earth and my wondering whether I was ready. Since then, I have preached in the mountains, valleys, and cities of Peru and America that Jesus is coming, and I have listened to my voice proclaiming this biblical truth. However, the reality is that I am getting older day by day, and He still has not come. Is this something that we expect with no time framing? The answer is a definite "no"! "Hope deferred makes the heart sick" (Prov 13:12). It is possible that many of us are losing our faith because of apparent tardiness, but His return is guaranteed. He will come again in His time, not ours. The prophecies of Matt 24, Mark 13, and Luke 21 are being accomplished before our eyes. The book of Daniel (7th to 6th centuries BCE), for example, give us just a glimpse of the living reality that we baptized with the name of modern technology: "But thou Daniel, shut up the words, and seal the book, even to the time of the end: many shall run to and fro, and knowledge shall be increased" (Dan 12:4). No Baby Boomer ever imagined in his or her youth the things that we see, use, and enjoy at the present time. God has His own time that is neither slow nor fast. This time is in His hand and when He is ready, we will see Him coming in glory and majesty. We certainly expect that all the current world commotions and unspeakable situations will be resolved with His Second Coming.

If we observe the wonderful universe created by God, we see that it is entirely an example of order; nothing is left to the last minute or to chance. Planets have to follow their orbits; the Sun has to radiate enough energy to keep us warm, but not burn; the oxygen has to remain stable in order for living creatures on earth to complete their cycle. God is amazing, and He did everything to show His supreme love to us. "The heavens declare the glory of God; and the firmament shewed knowledge" (Ps 19:1). Jesus' first coming was scheduled, and His second coming will also be scheduled.

According to Matthew, Jesus foretold that "this gospel of the kingdom will be preached in the whole world as a testimony to all nations, and then the end will come" (Matt 24:14 NIV). At the same time, the Scriptures made another point crystal clear: "But of the day and hour knoweth no man, no, not the angels of heaven, but my Father only" (Matt 24:36). Thus, if we have a God of order who is goal-oriented and has a plan, a chaplain, as an obedient servant, has to work in the same frame, with a concrete Road Map Plan (RMP), Stages of Changes (SOC) that are accurately evaluated, and a regular Quality of Life assessment (QOL) for every person/patient who was assigned to his or her intervention.

It is very clear that a good assessment will provide a tool for other things to be done. For example, Village and Piedmont (2013) found that "the women reported that they attend church more often than men" (p. 28). Research in the social-scientific study of religion is important. "Spirituality is understood to be one important construct in the creation of meaning in the lives of human beings" (Morris, 2013, para. 1).

This is the reason that RPCCC spent time and resources in creating a good tool of assessment with the capability to cover the basic spiritual needs of every patient admitted. Every year bereavement and grief education are promoted; an entire Pastoral Care Week is planned that ends with a luncheon for members of the pastoral care staff, clergy consultants, and Roswell Park staff to hear from patients how faith and culture carried them through the cancer journey. (Lenegan, 2018).

A time of breathing fresh air for the staff is vital. They should constantly remember how certain it is that spiritual endeavors take their toll. A chaplain's activities in the hospital are classified among the hazardous professions like other psychological matters. This is the major reason that hospitals promote Pastoral Care Team retreats, among other activities.

Direct impacts on the survivors also form part of the whole approach in serving the patients and families. Dedicated and serious spiritual care providers are concerned not just about providing support for the patients, but also for the families. The Pediatric Remembrance Service and the Fall Remembrance Service are also planned with great anticipation. They are really moments of closeness to the Lord. Family members and friends declare to the entire community that the family members, although no longer physically present, their presence and memories will last forever. I do not want to neglect mentioning the Tree of Hope Event, the Survivorship and Wellness Clinic, participation in the WNY End of Life committee, and the very notorious Life Recorded Program that gives patients and families valuables memories to treasure. According to Rabbi Eilberg (2000), the time of dying still has to be planned:

Try to remember to be gentle with yourself. You need to take breaks —meaningful breaks that can bring you rest, refreshment, and distraction. You need help because no one in the world can do this alone. You need other loved ones who can listen and support you because you may need to cry and rage. Your presence with your loved one can make a profound difference and his or her experience of the end of life. But you must take care yourself, too, in order to offer the best of yourself to your loved one. (pp. 5-6)

There is no time to be careless. When working in chaplaincy, more dedication, care, and preventive measures need to be put in place; as a consequence, more heavenly results will be harvested. "Although ongoing controversy about whether faith and spirituality should play a role in health care and back to the many ways that these powerful forces already function in healthcare today" (Cadge, 2012, para. 2). The results that we will see immediately impact the life of the patient, enhance his hope, and lessen his pain. A little mistake can cost the spiritual death of the patient and unnecessary pain, and we need to avoid this. We chaplains need to see ourselves working like surgeons and physicians, doing our best to save the life of the patient. Death is not in the mind of the surgical team. This must also be the rule in spiritual care. You probably remember the story of the Trojan Horse, as told in The Odyssey by Homer and in

The Aeneid by Virgil. In 1184 BC, there was an ancient city-state called Troy on the coast of Turkey, across the sea from Sparta. At one time, Troy and the other Greek city-states were quite good friends. But times changed.

The city of Troy was protected by high walls around the land, some over 20 feet high. There were gates in the wall to let the right people in and out and it provided a great defense for the people of Troy. Trojan warriors were stationed atop the walls, which provided a relatively safe place to stand guard and defend. The vantage point was perfect for soldiers to rain down arrows on any unfortunate enemy below who tried to break into the city. Greek warriors had been trying to breach these impenetrable walls for nearly ten years. The Greeks could not find a way in, and the Trojans did not seem able to drive the Greeks away. Finally, the mighty Greek general Odysseus, devised an incredible plan of attack. His strategy was to build a beautiful, enormous wooden horse as a gift to the Trojan people of "admitted defeat" and leave it outside the gate. As they did this, the entire Greek army then made the Trojans believe that they left Troy in defeat. The horse was hollow and thirty men were hiding inside. As the Greek warriors sailed away, the people of Troy rushed outside, cheering. They dragged the horse inside the city gates to keep it on display as a trophy celebrating their win, which is just what the Greek general thought they would do—gloat. That night, while the Trojan people were sleeping, the men hiding inside the wooden horse climbed out and opened the gates from withing the city. The waiting Greek army entered Troy, and that was the end of Troy (Donn & Martin, 2020, paras. 5-6). Just one careless moment brought the fall of the entire city. This is to say that patients are certainly more valued that an entire city. There are souls God appointed to you for your care and dedication, and He will request a detailed account. Matthew emphasized it when he said, "His Lord said unto him, well done, good and faithful servant; thou hast been faithful over a few things, I will make thee ruler over many things: enter in the joy of the Lord" (Matt 25:23).

Matthew 7:24-27 shows the reality of two men who decided to build a house. One used knowledge, assessment, planning, and common sense, and the other just made his building in a way that could not resist the furious winds and rain that were common in the time of Jesus. Those two individuals had a good plan to build a house. Both of them had the resources, the idea, and the desire. However, only one made a good assessment before building and the consequences were predictable. One the builders really reached his goal for his family, while the other, once again, faced failure and disappointment. I can imagine these two individuals very excitedly wanting to provide permanent shelter for their families instead of moving every time, which would be a really painful activity. Thus, they decided to build something stable, secure, and comfortable. I lived like that for more than ten years. More than once, I had to move during the crude winter season, and it is no fun moving in the winter when you live on the Canadian border. It only adds to the already painful action of moving.

When I finally built my own house, it was a big celebration for the entire family. I actually invited the mayor of the city, the media, and the neighbors to celebrate my success. No more moving, no more receiving directions from landlords about how to care for their property, freedom to leave and enter at any time, lodging for family and friends coming to visit me without asking permission or time-frame. Many things that we learned in the process of building a house was a significant experience that changes the life of a person and the entire family forever. Owning a house is really an American dream, but in my case, it required sitting down with my wife and going through the basic process of planning and assessment. It required selecting the bank that would support our plan, the real state contractor, and the location for the house, the neighborhood where the children would grow up, and even provision for a parking lot where our future sons-in-law would park their cars. Woodley (2011) remembered this story:

A "neighbor, an older professor who sports a plush white goatee, is one of the nicest atheists I've ever met. As we were cordially chatting in his backyard one day, I noticed his shed and exclaimed, "Wow, that's a great-looking shed. Who built it for you?' Puffing out his chest a bit, he said, "Why, thank you. I built it myself—from scratch of course." "That's amazing," I said. "How did you figure out how to do that?" "It's pretty simple," he told me. "First, you read books on shed-building. And then, you build yourself a shed. But there's one very important step between those two steps: you make a decision. You have to decide that you will build the shed. That's the most important step: make a decision. There is no other way, my friend. Once you make that decision the shed will get done." (p. 93).

Everything will be on the pathway to success when the idea is planned, programmed, and acted upon. Matthew has good examples of things that push us to move from the accidental situation to the planned materialization of dreams. At first glance, the wide way, the false prophets, the phony faith, and the house built on the sand all look good and feel right. After all, what is wrong with the implied profession of Matt 7:22? By calling Jesus, "Lord, Lord," these people seem to espouse doctrinal correctness. They could most likely sign the statement of faith that guides most evangelical churches. They have also engaged in successful and impressive ministries for Jesus— prophesying in his name, casting out demons, and performing miracles.

On the level of the Q parable, the obvious background picture is a feast (δεῖπνον) which a householder prepared, probably for his friends and acquaintances. The NT has already provided a similar account of the δεῖπνον which Herod made for the great and mighty in his kingdom (cf. Mark 6:21). However, surprisingly, all the prospective guests in our present parable failed to honor the invitation to attend the feast. This is an extraordinary twist to the story that gave way to the tensions that developed between the householder and his invited guests. Therefore, the first problem that confronts any attempt to give the parable a realistic bent is the nature of invitations to feasts in antiquity (Onyenali, 2013, p. 174).

Another parable that clearly depicts the need for previous assessment in order to get fruits is the parable of the Sower. It is obvious that preparation and selection of the soil play a big role in this process. No farmer has the good sense to expect a decent harvest when the soil has not been prepared. Farmers in Western New York still need to know other factors like climate, kind of seeds, soil texture, and preparation before a snow storm ruins their expected harvest. We see the same thing in reference to the parable of the two builders; the disastrous results came because of a clear lack of perception, seriousness in the assignments, having things planned with realistic results, and so on. The process of sowing in Mark 4:1-25 deserves more study because it can easily be compared with the assessment care needed in order to get results. Hospitals working with terminal patients assigned to the Palliative Care Team need to know, prior to any intervention, the kind of soil (heart, mind) they have before them. Like soil preparation in a real agricultural setting, we must be sure that nothing interferes with the healthy growth of the seed (rocks, bushes, environment, pests, rodents, etc.).

In terms of pastoral care, seeds are the resources available in the Pastoral Care Department in order to provide the spiritual healing process of the patient. The first resources are the personal preparation of the chaplain, knowledge of the resources available in the pastoral care office, the list of denominational volunteers approved and authorized to supply any request from the patient, and the spiritual and intellectual preparation of the visitor. Looks incredible but still the words we use when visiting patients is so important. That is the reason why Kunner (1999) said,

Through their personal stories, they develop a new framework for the stages of illness and an accompanying language with which to discuss it. Instead of addressing illness as combat with victims and survivors, theirs is a language of relationship, spirit, and integration. (para. 1).

The Roswell Park Comprehensive Cancer Center is rich in human and material resources. Most of the religious denominations are represented in the hospital. Thus, there is a large amount of resources that include written and audio, materials in various languages, religious objects, and other tangible items that can be provided free of charge for every request. Hospitals are stressful places for individuals. If the patient is in really bad condition, the time to rest is minimal. How many times have I had to write in my patient notes that "he/she was not visited because he/she was sleeping"? This is valuable time for the patient and needs to be respected. Patients are allowed to refuse a chaplain's visit, and that is recorded as Do Not Visit (DNV) on the daily file sheet.

If we want to reduce the statistics of suicide in the American population every year,

moving our public health-oriented suicide prevention efforts forward requires visionary leadership, honest appraisal of our past successes and failures, consensus building following meaningful debate and deliberation, engagement of all relevant stakeholders including patients and families, and active engagement in relevant communities. It is tragic that each year in America, 38,000 die by suicide; there is a recent spike in the rates of suicide in young veterans; and rates of suicidal behavior among lesbian, gay, bisexual, transgender, queer and questioning youth are frighteningly high in part due to bullying. These are numbers that we must—and we can—reduce. (Kaslow, 2014, p. 5)

The question is how we can slow down the trend of these tragic events? One option is by providing training to trainees and psychologists on suicide assessment and treatment, training community members as gatekeepers for identifying and "referring those at risk and creating, assessing and disseminating programs that have a broad impact" (Kaslow, 2014, p. 5). Thus, we need to remember that Jesus never sent His disciples to do His work without previous education, training, and specific guidance. Later on, His church did the same, for example, from the very beginning of what was to become the early church when the Lord selected His apostles (Dörnbrak, 2020). White (1911) said:

These men He purposed to train and educate as the leaders of His church. They in turn were to educate others and send them out with the gospel message. That they might have success in their work they were to be given the power of the Holy Spirit. Not by human might or human wisdom was the gospel to be proclaimed, but by the power of God. For three years and a half the disciples were under the instruction of the greatest Teacher the world has ever known. By personal contact and association, Christ trained them for His service. Day by day they walked and talked with Him, hearing His words of cheer to the weary and heavy-laden, and seeing the manifestation of His power in behalf of the sick and the afflicted. (p. 17)

Sowing the seeds of hope and peace are skillful assignments because waves of hope spread out.

Chaplains need to be educated and masterful in this ability. As Piotrowski (2017) pointed out about the end of life, "chaplains can be the catalyst in helping individuals and their families prepare for a good death" (p. 13). Otherwise, it will be a painful experience for the patient, adds to the difficult transition that is already taking place. In the secular such as mental health, professionals are constantly learning and innovating their skills to give patients the best they can:

Recovery as a social justice framework addresses how people who experience mental illness can increase being active agents to assist in improving their quality of life. Similarly, co-operative inquiry challenges the power imbalances that exist among marginalized and vulnerable groups by seeking to create relevant platforms for equality. (Lith, 2014, p. 179)

Adventist Chaplaincy Ministries (my endorser) requires a minimum of 30 credit hours of continuing education in chaplaincy per year in order to be endorsed. The Roswell Park Comprehensive Cancer Center provides two workshops per year of full-day training for chaplains and pastoral care supporters. In almost all areas of the science, workers need to comply with this requirement. Think how a non-trained visitor could provide spiritual support to an atheist patient who is in the same room with the mother, an active member of the Buddhist community; the father, a former Roman Catholic member, but who is now an active member of the Gnostic community; and an older brother who is an active member of a Protestant church in the area. This is a very challenging situation for a non-trained visitor. Every patient also has his/her own worldview with numerous ways of seeing medical treatment as some kind of necessary threat; this is especially true for those who have a background of using what was previously alternative medicine.

Complementary and alternative medicine (CAM) has emerged as a prevalent alternative treatment option for many individuals. In 2007, the National Health Interview Survey from the National Institutes of Health found that 38% of adults and 12% of children in the United States used some form of CAM. (1) The high prevalence of CAM use suggests that we need to define more adequately what major CAM categories exist in the United State. (Brown, 2013, para. 1)

The importance of trained visitors/chaplains at Roswell is so important.

The Pastoral Care Department invests time and material resources every year and provides courses of preparation for prospective visits which are scheduled on a yearly basis in order to make sure this important matter is. In addition, applicants who wish to be spiritual visitors must sign a responsibility compliance form before having any contact with our patients. We need to remember that every patient assigned by the Pastoral Care Director is a divine appointment. There is a specific purpose in that appointment. This commission, on occasion, could become just a listening presence. Patients just need to be heard with no interruptions and with no other opinions. The sacred moments spent with the patient is not for the gratification of the chaplain's ego, intellectual display of intelligence or a professional opportunity to develop skills. It is not the time to preach a sermon or even to think about a Bible study.

No, all the time is for the patients; my time is their time, and it needs to be respected deeply. In the Bible are numerous occasions where an apparently simple encounter was not an accident, but God's commission, scheduled to do his work (Acts 8:26-35, 35-38). If this is so, every visit will be a chaplain's commitment to bring hope and encouragement to the patient. As a general rule, not every patient will be able to accept an offer of prayer. In my own experience, I found ministers (pastors, priests, nuns, etc.) who are in hospital beds respond negatively to me about an offer of prayer. In the Senate, for example, Chaplain Barry Black offers prayers every day, but also acts as spiritual advisor and counselor that is also important (United States Senate, 2020). Patients, in general, need the presence of the chaplain and they have to be able to open their hearts to the presence of the spiritual provider, but not everyone will accept an inflexible agenda. Cultural issues must be understood. From the moment he/she steps into the room of the patient, in a matter of seconds, the chaplain must take everything into account. When we consider the life and ministry of Jesus, we must observe a clear distinction between his thinking, ideals, principles, and planning on one side and the way he accomplished this purposes on the other. In His day-to-day life and ministry, He identified Himself with Jewish culture, just as the Old Testament predicted of the Messiah. But the impact of His incarnation was universally applicable. Through His death and Resurrection. He would bear the sins of the world (Schantz, 2015, p. 59).

There are no insignificant details when chaplain is in the sacred realm of a patient. Unobserved cultural issues are can become big barriers to performing a fair intervention. I really understand why Roswell Park Comprehensive Cancer Center always has a chaplain for the major spiritual backgrounds of admitted patients: Roman Catholic and Protestants. Both have full-time chaplains working at the same time in the hospital. In the realm of Christianity, Catholics and Protestants explain justification very differently. According to Canon Law in the Catholic Church, the clergy can directly justify the repentant parishioner using the obligation of confession. We, as a Protestants, do not believe that. Members of the clergy can listen to members of the church, counsel them, provide scriptural support, but the one who forgives sinner is only God. Protestants do not believe in human intercessors.

For example, when rehabilitation counselors approach the cultural perception of resilience, they know an exploration of the culturally based differences in resilience is useful in light of the discrepancy that exists in how cultures interpret trauma. The manner in which emotions are expressed can serve as an indicator of resilience following a trauma. Somatization is another common method of processing negative emotions in cultures that do not approve of the verbal communication of strong emotions. Somatization has historically been judged to be problematic and dysfunctional in Western medicine. (Buse, Burker, & Bernacchio, 2013, para. 1)

There are enough reasons why Beth Lenegan prepared interfaith prayers booklet that show exactly how the major religions in the world view intercessory prayer offered by the chaplain:

Judaism: "O Lord my God, I cried unto thee, and thou has healed me"; Christianity: "The prayer of faith shall save the sick, and the Lord shall raise them up"; Islam: "When I am ill, it is He Who cures me"" Hinduism: "I free thee from all evil and disease, and unite thee with life"; Zoroastrianism: "My name is the bestower of health; my name is the best bestower of health"; Sikhism: "The love of the Lord is the healing remedy; the name of the Lord is the healing remedy"; Baha'i Faith: "Thy mercy to me is my healing and my succor in both this world and the world to come"; and Buddhism: "Health is the greatest gift; Contentment is the greatest wealth." (Lenegan & Clearence, 2015, p. 33)

For example, the approach for a Hindu patient is totally different than for a Muslim patient.

While there is evidence that African Americans find spiritual resources helpful, there is also evidence that they experience salient spiritual distress, and that this may affect their recovery from trauma. It seems that African American patients receive greater benefit when chaplains intervene spiritually than other members of the community. Very often they openly display a great sense of gratitude and gladness and are likely to give feedback when required.

Given these cultural considerations, Building Spiritual Strength (BSS) is an 8-session, spiritually integrated group intervention designed to address religious strain and enhance religious meaning making for military trauma survivors. It is based upon empirical research on the relationship between spirituality and adjustment to trauma. To assess the intervention's effectiveness, veterans with histories of trauma who volunteered for the study were randomly assigned to a BSS group (n = 26) or a wait-list control group (n = 28). BSS participants showed statistically significant reductions in PTSD symptoms based on self-report measures as compared with those in a wait-list control condition. Further research on spiritually integrated interventions for trauma survivors is warranted. (Harris et al., 2011, p. 425)

The openness and skill of the visitor will make a difference. Jesus was very multiculturally oriented in His interactions because one soul was always so valuable for Him. The case of the Samaritan woman explains this: "The Samaritan woman was alert, was well-informed about the history of her people, and she asked intelligent questions" (Schantz, 2015, p. 65). The same tactic and knowledge are also found in the case of the Roman army officer: "The centurion understood and respected Jewish religious sensitivities...Jesus pointed out that the centurion was a prototype of the great day when people from all over the world join the Jewish patriarchs at the Messianic banquet" (Schantz, 2015, p. 6). For example, with patients who are Bible- oriented, "one sentence of the Scripture is of more value than ten thousand of man's ideas or arguments" (White, 1923, p. 253). The chaplain needs to listen to the Word of God to give a sensitive and helpful statement.

I remember that on one occasion, I found a Jewish patient in my list of visitations. Before I entered the room, I found the Jewish

Prayer (from the Torah) to say for him; I selected the right brochure to give him during visit; I was ready to interact with him about how Jews celebrate a Season of Miracles throughout the year because in the Jewish calendar, the time around Hanukkah—when we in North America know the reality of winter—is usually considered the season of miracles.

Chanukah or Hanukkah, is the eight-day festival of light, which begins on the eve of the 25th of the Jewish month of Kislev, to celebrate the triumph of light over darkness, spirituality over materiality, and of purity over adulteration. Mostly, and according to Judaism, it celebrates the fact that God can make miracles for those who stand up for truth and justice. The Menorah (nine-branched chandelier) lighting symbolizes chasing away forces of darkness, which the faithful Jews did with swords, but in this case with light. (Gómez, 2019, para. 1)

When I entered the room, I found that the patient was a smiling gentleman musician and he really wanted to talk about his musical instruments and personal achievements. A big organ had been set up in the room and many books were on it. He was inclined to talk about music and the entire world situation during the entire visit. He seemed very excited during the visit. When I asked about his religious background, he told me that he was a Jew, but had never visited a synagogue in his life. This response changed everything I had prepared. I never had the opportunity to open my previously selected prayers and share my Jewish brochures. not just he not showed interest but also the medical team came (scheduled time of observation) to the room and decided to start working with the patient. This was the end of my visitation. I left the room before I even open my book of prayers and share my brochure and even I had no opportunity to talk about the Jewish season of miracles.

We always need to remember who we are and whom we are visiting. There is a big difference between visiting a long-term patient and one who was recently diagnosed with cancer. Ghoshal, Miriyala, Elangovan, & Rai (2016) found that 89 patients participated in this study, of which only 19 could fill the questionnaire on their own. Anxiety was the most common symptom (97.8%) followed by depression (89.9%), tiredness (89.9%), and pain (86.5%). The treating physicians recorded pain in 83.1%, whereas the other symptoms were either not documented or grossly underreported. Anxiety was documented in 3/87 patients, but depression was not documented in any. Tiredness was documented in 12/80 patients, and loss of appetite in 54/77 patients mentioning them in the questionnaire. Significant statistical correlation could be seen between the presence of pain, anxiety, depression, tiredness, and loss of appetite in the patients. (p. 326)

A skilled chaplain is always needed.

Latino patients are one of my assignments at Roswell Park Comprehensive Cancer Center and they need to be cared for while taking into account their needs and culture that are so different from others. We do not need to be "enhanced stressors" for those who already have their "plates full." I found a sad scenario in another hospital. An elderly immigrant male was tied to the bed because he was trying to express what he needed, but nobody understood. Thus, he tried to get out of his bed and fell down. The doctor's solution was to tie him down. When I arrived in the room and asked the patient what the problem was, he explained that he needed to go bathroom. Because he had never been in a hospital before, he did not know that he had been given adult Pampers so he did not need to go to the bathroom. This situation added stress for this patient and could be detrimental to his recovery. For example, Claudia Medina from Louisiana State University stated, "Explanations for culture-bound syndromes are seen as reactions to trauma. People within any cultural group are not homogeneous, even though they may hold many beliefs, practices, and institutions in common. Messages and materials must respect the variations within." She also added, "Understanding how social, structural, psychological, and cultural factors affect physical health and being sensitive to these factors can make an important difference in health outcomes" (Medina, 2020, para. 2). This is also understood under the lenses of the people who have a language barrier. You can imagine as a chaplain trying to perform your palliative care assessment, but the patient needs an interpreter and the interpreter has no clinical preparation. This is also crucial. Ingvarsdotter, Johnsdotter, and Ostman (2012) noted the following in her research: "Choosing an interpreter is one of the main tasks in planning field interview and various recommendations have been given in this regard" (p. 35). There are many interpreters who have no idea about mental health or notions of oncology, and this can absolutely bias the results of the assessment.

The same sensitivity must be observed when questions arise during visits. Years ago, when I was visiting a 64-year-old Roman Catholic patient, I found the room filled with family members. On the Census Sheet Report was the indication that he was an End of Life Patient (EOL). After I introduced myself to everyone, the first question from the patient was where he would go when died, to heaven or to hell. There was silence in the room as everyone waited for my answer. All the relatives were expecting the right answer from my perspective. I replied that only God could answer that question because God gives salvation, and the chaplain is not there to decide the final destination of each individual. However, I also explained to the patient and the relatives that in most cases, we decide where we want to go, that salvation is a personal decision. I explained that God had already accomplished His plan of salvation and wants everyone to be saved, but that He does not force people to make one decision or another. Thank God the patient and the relatives in the room seemed pleased by the answer. This is confirmed by the research of the Karoliska Institute: "Results confirm that reciprocity is fundamental for relationships, and that recognizing the individual entails personal involvement. The participants describe a struggle and recognizing this struggle may help the professional to achieve a deeper understanding of the individual" (Adnoy, Sundfor, Karlsson, Raholm, & Arman, 2012, p. 357).

There is another interesting question I find very common among patients who have no other option than to spend their last days at home. That question concerns the method of burial. They ask me about my opinion on cremation. When possible, I first try to find out their opinions. I consider this necessary.

Modern missiology applies the term contextualization to Paul mission methods stated here. Contextualization is defined as an attempt to communicate the Gospel in word and deed and to establish the church in ways that make sense to people's needs and penetrates their worldview, thus allowing them to follow Christ and remain within their own culture. (Schantz, 2015, p. 94)

The case of a patient who was sedated and intubated for more than two months was interesting. The patient's niece was an infallible presence in her aunt's room. The patient was an African American woman and a former missionary. The doctor's panel (ethical committee) recommendation was that the patient needed to have the machinery deactivated in order to allow the natural process of healing or physical degradation. When the doctors called to consult with the family concerning this issue, one of the family members rejected the plan, adding that her aunt would need more time before getting off the respiratory and tubing machines. This caused a tense relationship between the family members and the medical team. Various questions were posed, but one in particular needed to be answered. What kind of beliefs did the family have? Talking with the niece who was always present in the room, the chaplain discovered that she was also a physician working at a sister hospital in the community. She had never disclosed this information except to the chaplain; she knew exactly what was happening with her aunt. The other point that came to light after much discussion was that the patient's niece believed in miracles. She was expecting a miracle and that it would come in God's time. In fact, before the week ended, the patient woke up. In a couple of weeks, she started speaking and moving her extremities. At the end of a month, she left the intensive care unit and was placed in a rehabilitation room and was discharged during the following month. Things like that sometimes challenge the medical team and the chaplain's intervention is necessary to clarify possible misunderstanding. Here we understand that "providing spiritual care is about tapping into the concept of spirituality: core meaning, deepest life meaning, hope and connectedness" (MacKinlay & Trevitt, 2007, p. 74).

Clinical application

The concept of the relation of sickness and body has a high impact in understanding a patient's needs when he/she is hospitalized. For example traditional Chinese medicine (TCM) recognizes the unity that exists between physical body (e.g., organ physiological process) and the mind (e.g., emotions, thoughts) and this constant interplay between the mind and body is important when considering the methods and practices that facilitate healing. (Buse et al., 2014, para. 1)

The sacredness of the body is not viewed in the same way; it varies from culture to culture. For example, this is the reason why some scholars struggle with the writings of Hillel when he said that death in childbirth is like punishment "because they are not careful regarding the laws of niddah (ritual and sexual purity), challah (the tithing of dough to a priest), and the kindling of the Sabbath candle" (Kirsch, 2012, para. 3). He continued, Why should failing to light a Sabbath candle deserve the death penalty? "Because the soul that I have placed within you," God might reply, "is called a candle" (in the Book of Proverbs: "The candle of God is man's soul"). And why, in particular, should it be death in childbirth that God inflicts? "Because," says Rava, "When the ox has fallen, sharpen the knife": in other words, childbirth is a time when a woman is already vulnerable to death, just as a fallen ox is vulnerable to slaughter. (para. 3)

Jesus' teachings always found that we need to speak the "right word at the right time" (White, 1930, p. 227). What I found during my routine visits at Roswell Park was that sometimes it is not the patient who rejects the presence of a chaplain, but the family. Other times, the opposite takes place. Thus, in order to know exactly what and where the urgent need is, masterful skill is necessary. "The lack of background information about the characteristics and health status of the careers can be a major limitation" (Kajiwara, Kako, & Miyashita, 2019, para. 3). God even led the trumpeters of Zion; similarly, the sacredness of the chaplain's mission is so high that the enemy is ever ready to mislead him. There is a mission that needs to be accomplished in every hospital setting, but without the anointing of the Holy Spirit, this is impossible, and souls perish without hope. The words of the minister during a patient visit must be carefully chosen. Some can lead to hope, peace, and encouragement, but others can lead to hopelessness and despair. White (1892) commented that the way some pastors behave is very important.

I saw that ministers, as well as people, have warfare before them to resist Satan. The professed minister of Christ is in a fearful position when serving the purposes of the tempter, by listening to his whisperings, and letting him captivate the mind and guide the thoughts. The minister's most grievous sin in the sight of God is talking about his unbelief, and drawing other minds into the same dark channel, thus suffering Satan to carry out a twofold purpose in tempting him. He unsettles the mind of the one whose course has encouraged his temptations, and then leads that one to unsettle the minds of many. It is time that the watchmen upon the walls of Zion understood the responsibility and sacredness of their mission. They should feel that a woe is upon them if they do not perform the work which God has committed to them. If they become unfaithful, they are endangering the safety of the flock of God, endangering the cause of truth, and exposing it to the ridicule of our enemies. O what a work is this! It will surely meet its reward. Some ministers, as well as people, need converting. They need to be torn to pieces, and made over new. Their work among the churches is worse than lost, and in their present weak, tottering condition, it would be more pleasing to God for them to cease their efforts to help others, and labor with their hands until they are converted. Then they could strengthen their brethren. (p. 120)

Every aspect related to a patient is very important and must be treated with delicateness. "The effects of cancer vary from couple to couple. For some couples, facing the challenges of cancer together strengthens their relationship. For others, the stress of cancer may create new problems and worsen existing problems" (Asco, 2019, para. 1). "Three themes emerged: a sense of assuming a different identity as the disease challenged abilities, the experience of social isolation with fear of dependence and barriers the participants encountered acting as obstacles to coping, adapting and accessing treatments" (Ellison, Gask, Bakerly, & Roberts, 2012, p. 308). My wife Mary, for example, likes gardening. She really enjoys seeing her roses, lilies, and vegetables grow. Every summer, she is concerned about the preparation of the soil, about buying the right soil, fertilizer, fences, and so on for the garden in our backyard. She loves planting, caring for her plants, and discussing with other gardeners what she needs to do to grow bigger tomatoes or how to get her watermelon plants to produce fruit. She is a passionate gardener, but still needs to learn many techniques to hone her skills. In the parable of the sower, we find the one who eagerly wanted to see his plants bear fruit. He tried many kinds of soils and still got negative results. Chaplains never skip or neglect an individual patient. Everyone is worthy of attention and care, but without enough experience, it can be devastating for the sower and for the seeds. If the sower never grows to the point of maturity, the fruits themselves will lack growth. My wife has to be intentional about how to garden. Fortunately, there are many magazines in the store workshops during the summer that she can attend, TV demonstrations, and internet gardening clubs. Education is vital in gardening, but still more vital for visiting a patient in the hospital. Social justice is partly our responsibility. Other countries like the United Kingdom unite efforts to address mental health issues: "The survey identified two clusters of research topics as future priorities for the social research agenda: the first is social inclusion/social capital and social networks, and the second is resilience and recovery" (Gould, Huxley, & Tew, 2007, p. 179). In the same manner, chaplains need to unite all resources to help the palliative community.

Many theologians or seminarians believe that because of their title or diploma, they are ready to be chaplains. However, this is not true. I know chaplains who, instead of reading and expanding their knowledge about chaplaincy, now spend their time reading other kinds of literature out of the scope of chaplaincy. This is a bad idea. Extra training is required. There are enormous differences between pastoring a church congregation and pastoring a patient in the hospital. The environment of the church is not the same as the environment of the hospital. Church pastors are usually geared toward Bible studies and sermons. When they visit a hospital, they have in mind how to evangelize that person, how to convert him or her. Most pastors believe that if they do not baptize an individual, their work is incomplete. Proselytizing is discordant in a hospital setting. Therefore, pastors need to be trained to become chaplains. There is a wider perception of the labor of ministry in hospitals than in churches. In some areas of the world, chaplains are seen as deserters of the true pastoral ministry. Of course, this is the fruit of ignorance rather than knowledge.

This is their major concern. It has been said that every chaplain is a pastor, but not every pastor is a chaplain. There is a great difference. While the sower wanted to have fruits as a result of his work, chaplains will also receive double the joy when the ministry is well done. Their ministry fills their hearts with a heavenly feeling when the work is done correctly, but heaven also erupts with joy that is the result of good ministry. Trained chaplains, well-prepared ministers, will never surrender under adverse circumstances. What kept Jesus on the cross, bleeding and suffering unimaginable pain was what He looked forward to: the salvation of all humanity, his followers walking with him in the New Canaan, and the hope of redemption for humanity. Sowing is not an easy task. The sower in the parable had a lot of disappointments, but he persisted and found the perfect soil for his task. The sower sowed his seed in every type of ground; he never neglected one soil.

The chaplain's commitment is to serve all. If he has preferences, he is not living up to the mandate of his ministry. Contrary to the practice of psychology, a counselor or a psychiatrist can decide who to serve or not to serve. He has to make that decision. In chaplaincy, there is no such decision. A sick person is God's creation and must be cared for. Every heart needs to be prepared to receive the seeds of truth; otherwise, it will be a complete disappointment for both the minister and the person who is the focus of that ministry. The presence of the Holy Spirit is vital at every visit. The successful visit is not merely human skills displayed, but a minister surrendered to the Lord. The whole universe is witness to the work being done. Every chaplain has been called to do his ministry with passion, love, and knowledge, but also to keep in mind these words: "Well done, good and faithful servant; you have been faithful over a few things, I will make you ruler over many things. Enter into the joy of your lord" (Matt 25:23).

It is true that we have to visit every patient entering the hospital, but we also need to understand that not everyone is ready to have a visit from a chaplain. That is the reason to request another "counselor" (the Holy Spirit) who will help us discern the real reason behind the rejection of a chaplain' visit. Many times, the patient explains why, and I have to listen carefully; other times, the patient cannot explain why, but just reacted when he or she saw you and the chaplain's observations must suffice. Sometimes it is clear to the chaplain because the patients say, "I don't need a visit." In this case, it is the patient's decision and needs to be honored. The most important thing is that the minister must never take the patient's reaction personally; we are their "important ally in providing religious and spiritual interventions for mental health patients" (Duru, 2016, para. 1).

There are many issues in people's lives that a visitor cannot see. Some of them mask other concerns. On one occasion, a lady was having treatment in the hospital because of her stage four cancer. Her daughter was also being treated for cancer on the floor below, and her husband was at home recovering from a car accident. I thanked God for the opportunity to visit this patient. Her tear-filled eyes and concerned words showed me what she was really experiencing at the time of my visit. We are called to understand these kinds of circumstances. The power of the Holy Spirit has to show us how to combine His wisdom with our experience. Spending time in prayer in the hospital chapel is so valuable in making wise decisions. Jesus was a great example. Before going into a spiritual encounter, He needed to gain power by bowing down in prayer. Gethsemane has to be the book and pathway for every true chaplain. Our hearts have to be filled with the Holy Spirit so that we become "rivers of living water" (John 7:38). Our assignment requires powerful spirituality, strong conviction, and total dependence on the Lord. When the disciples started doing their ministry while He was physically present, Jesus said, "Behold, I send you out as sheep in the midst of wolves. Therefore be wise as serpents and harmless as doves" (Matt 10:16). White (1946) commented:

Many souls are hungering for the bread of life. Their cry is, "Give me bread; do not give me a stone. It is bread that I want." Feed these perishing, starving souls. Let our minister's bear in mind that the strongest meat is not to be given to babes who know not the first principles of the truth as we believe it. In every age the Lord has had a special message for the people of that time; so we have a message for the people in this age. But while we have many things to say, we may be compelled to withhold some of them for a time, because the people are not prepared to receive them now. (p. 200)

Human Dignity (Genesis 3) Creation

From the beginning we can understand that creation of the human being was special in comparison with the creation of the other creatures. God just used a command to create everything else: "Let the waters abound with an abundance of living creatures, and let birds fly above the earth" (Gen 1:20) to create all the living creatures in the sea and birds flying from one side to the other and a similar command on the sixth day for the earth to bring forth all animals that moved along the ground. However, when the Lord planned to create mankind, he used different terminology: "Let us make man in Our image, according to Our likeness . . . So God created man in His own image, in the image of God He created him; male and female He created them" (Gen 1:26, 27). This is enough proof that when we deal with human beings, special rules need to be applied. They are made in the image of God; they are beings who have dignity, feelings, emotions, and desires that the chaplain needs to take into consideration regarding everything that is related to them. When they are in the hospital, they keep their royalty as children of the heavenly King; every single facet of this that they receive from conception, from creation, they receive from God. A visit from a chaplain must be seen as entering into a sacred place; there is a sanctuary that needs to be addressed and needs to be fulfilled with all the care that is worthy for God's handiwork. There is nothing acceptable in a job that sees humanity as less than the object of God commitment. In the Catholic arena concerning bioethics, we read:

Given the Catholic view that a person does not have the moral right to take serious risks to health, the likelihood of harm will set limits to participation in clinical trials. The deliberate use of deception in psychological or behavioral experiments is also problematic for those who take the view that deception is inherently wrong and cannot be justified by the beneficial results of a study. With respect to genetic research, the generally accepted principles that protect confidentiality, privacy, self- determination, justice and, ultimately, the dignity of the human person are compatible with Catholic health care ethics. The Church has always sought to embody our Savior's concern for the sick. (United States Conference of Catholic Bishops, 2009, para. 2)

Redemption

However, not only are we worthy to be treated with dignity because of our origin, but also because of the care God used after the fall. In His word, we find the most relevant summary of His love: "For God so loved the world that He gave His only begotten Son, that whoever believes in Him should not perish but have everlasting life" (John 3:16). There are two basic gifts that indebt us to God: creation and redemption. What a great honor for humankind to have such dignity provided by our Father God. Is this not enough reason to see every single patient with the title that he/she deserves? Chaplains around the world know these implications, and the way they approach a patient demonstrates how they understand the two aspects of God as Creator and Redeemer. In reference to a person's dying, Brennan (2014) mentioned that "memorialization, commemoration, and grieving is one recent trend in cultural expression regarding death and dying" (para. 3).

Historical review

From Genesis to Revelation, God expresses carefully the value and dignity of every one of His creatures. Free will was provided only to humankind as the crown of creation. No human deserves lesser recognition. The death of Jesus on the cross marked forever the deepest love of the Creator for His creatures. Chaplains are here to display in real time God's desire for people to know and experience this.

Ethical implications in the assessment

Assessment of the palliative care patient is vital. The World Health Organization (WHO) definition of palliative care is

> an approach that improves the quality of life of patients and their families facing the problems

associated with life-threatening illness, through the prevention and relief of suffering by means of early identification and impeccable assessment and treatment of pain and other problems, physical, psychosocial and spiritual. (Sharma, Varma, Anusha, & Bharti, 2013, p. 293)

This program is expanding and becoming more important every year. "Palliative care teams in hospitals have rapidly expanded to provide care for seriously ill patients irrespective of prognosis. To date, over two-thirds of all hospitals and over 85% of mid to large size hospitals report a palliative care team" (Morrison, 2013, p. 201). Organizations like the WHO do not just apply palliative care to adults, but also to children. The WHO Definition of Palliative Care (2013) states:

Palliative care for children represents a special, albeit closely related field to adult palliative care and is the active total care of the child's body, mind and spirit, and also involves giving support to the family. It begins when illness is diagnosed and continues regardless of whether or not a child receives treatment directed at the disease. Health providers must evaluate and alleviate a child's physical, psychological, and social distress. Effective palliative care requires a broad multidisciplinary approach that includes the family and makes use of available community resources; it can be successfully implemented even if resources are limited. It can be provided in tertiary care facilities, in community health centers and even in children's homes. (Downing et al., 2014, para. 3)

As I said earlier, a person lying in a hospital bed or any person we interact with has to be treated ethically. When we proceed to develop a spiritual assessment, many ethical points must be put into practice. "The most important ethical considerations are summarized as: Justice, autonomy, beneficence and non-maleficence according to the basic principles of medical ethics" (Stanford University, 2019, para. 2); there is no way to avoid these principles. Beauchamp and Childress (2012) from the Kennedy Institute of Ethics also stated that these considerations include moral principles of respect for autonomy (the obligation to respect the decision making capacities of autonomous persons); non-maleficence (the obligation to avoid causing harm); beneficence (obligations to provide benefits and to balance benefits against risks), and justice (obligations of fairness in the distribution of benefits and risks. (para. 2)

A real and serious spiritual assessment will honor these rules and, under all circumstances, avoid putting an extra load on the life of the patient who is barely overcoming situations that are unimaginable for a person who has never gone through the same situation. "When all clinicians strive to meet those needs, we can all look forward to the health and social benefits. Responding to ethical and justice issues in mental health care is an obligation for all of us" (Reid, 2016, p. 567). People with cancer have enough to bear. Chaplains and clinicians need to avoid putting more burdens on them. "Since people with progressive, life-limiting illnesses experience distress in many domains, effective care in this context often requires a comprehensive and interdisciplinary approach. Palliative care is now broadly recognized as an essential treatment model in this scenario" (Fairman & Irwin, 2014, p. 6).

Informed Consent

The Informed Consent Form is very important and needs to be reviewed by the person who is receiving any treatment, be it medical or for a research activity. I used the Informed Consent Form that was prepared especially for the purpose of the research and was also approved by the Institutional Review Boards of Roswell Park Comprehensive Cancer Center and Andrews University (see Appendix D). The process was a little lengthy, but at the end of the day, it was worthwhile for the participants. One of the reasons for having the informed consent is to create confidence and show that the work we are trying to perform is serious.

Liability

Since we are working with humans, every action we take is subject to liability.

Liability for damages associated with a research project is a concern of institutions executing agreements related to collaborations. It would not be possible to list all the instances in which liability may arise, but we can address some of them that have a reasonable potential of occurring. Lawsuits or financial claims can arise from negligence or other wrongdoing that may occur in the performance of the project work. We usually think of these damages as being related to personal injury or damage to equipment and/or facilities. (Office of Research Integrity, 2019, para. 2)

JCAHO Deliberations

The JCAHO makes recommendations every year to assure that service is reaches perfection. The Joint Commission on Accreditation of Healthcare Organizations is a private, not for profit organization established in 1951 to evaluate health care organizations that voluntarily seek accreditation. The Joint Commission evaluates and accredits more than 16,000 health care organizations in the United States, including 4,400 hospitals, more than 3,900 home care entities, and over 7,000 other health care organizations that provide behavioral health care, laboratory, ambulatory care, and long term care services. The Joint Commission also evaluates and accredits health plans and health care networks. It is governed by representatives from the American College of Physicians, the American College of Surgeons, the American Dental Association, the American Hospital Association, the American Medical Association, an at-large nursing representative, six public members, and the Joint Commission President. (U.S. Department of Health and Human Services, Office of Disease Prevention and Health Promotion, 2019, para. 3)

This organization advised the Roswell Park Comprehensive Cancer Center for the first time in the use of palliative care assessment to gather enough information from patients, either new admits or those who needed follow–ups. The JCAHO established the fact that the work of the chaplain is an intimate relationship with God's creation: a human being. We are indeed creatures molded by the hand of the Owner of the universe. He also prepared our first father Adam and our first mother Eve. From this perspective, we need to realize that human beings are worthy of dignity, respect, and freedom as their advice document explains. Another thing that caught my attention that religion and medicine were together at the beginning of the history of the human race. However, the advance of science and, I may add, the influence of the Greek philosophy led by Plato have created what they called a chasm between the two.

The JCAHO understands that we are not just physical bodies. We have a spiritual aspect along with the physical component. This is the premise where chaplains work especially since recent studies show that "82% of Americans believe in the healing power of personal prayer" (Levy, 2011, para. 2). It does not matter what one' s faith, religion, or label for that connection with God, or connection with the "Higher Power" may be; these are tremendous tools to help the person waiting for restoration. A long time ago, I discovered in my visitation list the name of lady who was in her 60s. She had been admitted to the hospital because of ovarian cancer. The only problem was that she spoke only Arabic. My director assigned me to find out what we could do for her in the spiritual arena. When I approached the room, I found her older son, an engineering professor at the University of Toronto, sitting beside his mother. When I greeted them, he immediately said that his mother only understood Arabic and he would be translating for her.

I immediately asked her the question about her faith, and she responded that she was a member of the Muslim community in Toronto, Canada. I thought this was the moment to ask whether she needed someone from her own faith community to give her spiritual support. She declined but added: "You can do it for me." It surprised me but gave me permission to try to do something new. I found in my electronic tools a Muslim Prayer for the sick which seemed to comfort her when repeated during the intervention. During the intervention, the JCAHO also requires chaplains to respond to the basic questions of all patients such as, "Why do I exist? Why I am ill? Will I die and what will happen to me when I die?" Based on what the spiritual assessment brings, chaplains need to present a plan of action and goals that will at least try to respond to these basic questions. On another occasion, a chaplain received an urgent call from the 5th floor of another hospital in the south part of the city. When chaplain arrived, he found that a Muslim woman had miscarried at eight months, the third baby in the family. The husband immediately allowed the chaplain to continue with the visit.

Many of the patients try to respond to these questions, but the problem is that they need help. Walking in the pathway of uncertainty leads to burn out. Many of them have pre-conceptions that bias their own self-understanding. As they try to respond to the question of why they are ill, some of them believe that the physical problem they have is a normal condition inherited form the family genes. However, if we analyze the response more closely, we do not find just one answer, but many. Others blame themselves for their situation and think they need to be punished in order to recover. This is the reason for the chaplain's presence, to help them really find the truth. Many of them simply block their restoration because of their own ideologies, and they have that right.

We must always understand the values of the human in exploring possibilities to decide for one treatment or another. This includes the chaplain's visit. If the patient simply rejects the visit, that decision must be cordially respected. It is his/her will. The patient has the right to be respected. The holistic approach will attend the total need of the person. We do not know what difficulties they are facing besides the cancer.

Death—lingering, unexpected, violent, or self- inflicted—and the loss of a relationship—to oneself or with a child, sibling, parent, mate, grandparent, or friend—give life to grief, together with the process by which each person fully encounters his or her grief. (Halamish & Hermoni, 2007, para. 2)

We are treating a human being who is not just physical or intellectual. There is the spiritual component that needs nutrition in the same way that we need to take care of our physical bodies. As professional chaplains, we are appointed to reinforce this concept. From the standpoint of legal issues, the consideration of the individual is very important, and chaplains are called to do the best in their call to duty:

> The element of duty is the legal obligation to exercise reasonable care under the circumstances, whether you are driving a car, building a bridge, or performing surgery. In the healthcare field, physicians owe a duty to their patients to exercise the level of skill and care that is provided by similar professionals under similar circumstances. (Harris, 2008, p. 209)

The holistic approach is required. The literature highlights the importance of the workplace culture that has to do with the spiritual needs of the staff members. I totally agree with this point. The staff members continually rely on the presence of the chaplain to face issues regarding patient care or relationships with the family. It is no doubt very stressful for the staff to deal with families who give them a hard time or at the passing of long-term patients with whom they had created a bond. Chaplains' help seemed vital for many medical teams.

I remember when one of the nurses approached me and asked me to talk to the older son of a dying mother. The son truly believed in the miracle of healing. When the medical team told him clearly that his mother was no longer treatable, his reaction was total denial, and he accused the staff of negligence. However, the reality was that his mother was in the fourth stage cancer and she was already brain dead with no possibility of recovery. Here was the time for intervention! Creating a safe environment between patients and families and working with the clinical staff is when chaplains are called to work. I would like to finish this summary by saying that professional chaplains act as mediators and reconcilers, functioning in the following ways for those who need a voice in the healthcare system: As advocates or "cultural brokers" between institutions and patients, family members, and staff Clarifying and interpreting institutional policies to patients, community clergy, and religious organizations Offering patients, family members and staff an emotionally and spiritually "safe" professionals from whom they seek counsel or guidance representing community issues and concerns to the organizations. (Association of Professional Chaplains, 2020, p. 7)

According to many American researchers, the use of palliative care in the life of a patient came as a result of an evolution from the sole care of ELP that was only to give the patient comfort during his last days:

> Palliative care began with a focus on the care of the dying. Dr. Cicely Saunders first articulated her ideas about modern hospice care in the late 1950s based on the careful observation of dying patients. She advocated that only an interdisciplinary team could relieve the "total pain" of a dying person in the context of his or her family, and the team concept is still at the core of palliative care. In the 1960s, a psychiatrist in the United States, Elisabeth Kübler-Ross, confronted fierce resistance to treating people at the end of life with respect, openness and honest communication. Her groundbreaking book, On Death and Dying, and charismatic presentations

revolutionized and humanized how dying patients were acknowledged and cared for. In 1974, Dr. Balfour Mount, a surgical oncologist at The Royal Victoria Hospital of McGill University in Montreal, Canada, coined the term palliative care to avoid the negative connotations of the word hospice in French culture, and introduced Dr. Saunders' innovations into academic teaching hospitals. He first demonstrated what it meant to provide holistic care for people with chronic or life-limiting diseases and their families who were experiencing physical, psychological, social, or spiritual distress. (LosCalzo, 2008, p. 465)

The care was extended in various fronts that include the family at the same time the care was expanded to the comfort, to the psychological area, social needs, pain care, and also the spiritual area of the patients and extended to the closest network. "Palliative care offers careful attention to pain and symptom management, added support for patient and families, and assistance with difficult medical decision making alongside any and desired medical treatments" (Quill & Miller, 2014, para. 3).

Modern Trends Regarding Palliative Spiritual Care Assessment

American Model

The major emphasis also changed from inpatient to outpatient status:

US palliative care is now conceptualized as patient- centered and family-centered care that optimizes quality of life by anticipating, preventing, and treating suffering. Palliative care is operationalized through effective management of pain and other distressing symptoms, while incorporating psychosocial and spiritual care with consideration of patient/family needs, preferences, values, beliefs, and culture. Palliative care is provided concurrently with all other appropriate treatments including those directed at cure and life prolongation by a team of physicians, nurses, social workers, chaplains, and other relevant healthcare professionals as needed. (Morrison, 2013, p. 201)

The role of the chaplain has been greatly valued, and now there are schools of medicine that promote palliative care studies, and physicians are very involved in this new area of medicine. Chaplains throughout the United States also receive extended training so they may serve much better as part of the palliative care team. Chaplains are called to assist them during visitations, re-assessments, pastoral consults, and to be nearby during family meetings. As chaplain, I play a big role on the palliative care team. In the past, this service was only offered to inpatients, but now this approach has changed.

Patients living in the community who are not hospice eligible have had few palliative care options available to them and very little palliative care is provided by generalists. The environment, however, is changing as the provisions of the PPACA provide fiscal and quality incentives to deliver palliative care outside of hospitals leading to the development of community palliative care models that include primary, secondary, and tertiary models of palliative care delivery. (Morrison, 2013, p. 201)

European Model

Palliative care (PC) that was developed in European countries had a major impact when they integrated various areas of care for individuals with life-threatening diseases. Much research has been done to demonstrate evidence-based plans to help patients, and the results are astounding. Eligible studies included those focusing on models of integrated PC for adult patients with cancer or another chronic disease (COPD, renal failure, heart failure, HIV, dementia or other types of neurological diseases), that are, in turn, consistent with the above- mentioned definitions of models and of integrated PC. Since our primary objective concerns the identification of evidence-based models, only those studies that empirically assessed the effectiveness of these models and provided relevant data were considered eligible. In particular, we considered randomized controlled trials (RCTs), quasi experimental studies, cohort studies, controlled before-and-after studies, observational studies and pilot evaluation studies whereas we excluded theoretical studies, audits, opinion-only studies in clinical case reports, editorials and letter. (Siouta et al., 2016, Selection criteria section, para. 3)

The interesting thing regarding European models of PC are still in progress. They are very attuned to how it is evolving and follow very closely the findings of the WHO.

According to the World Health Organization (WHO), Palliative Care (PC) aims to improve the quality of life of patients and families who face life-threatening illness, by providing pain and symptom relief, spiritual and psychosocial support from diagnosis to end of life care and bereavement. Caregivers of patients with advanced cancer often face physical, social, and emotional distress as well as spiritual pain. (Delgado et al., 2013, p. 455)

Further, the WHO recommends that PC becomes an integral part of healthcare and that all patients affected by a life threatening disease should have access to PC services. This statement is further supported by the European Association of Palliative Care and is also in agreement with the guidelines of the European Council towards the European Union (EU) Member States. (Siouta et al., 2016, Background section, paras. 1, 3)

Chapter reflections

- The Decision to be a Chaplain.
- Characteristics and preparation of a Chaplain.
- How important is Pastoral Care in a patient.
- What results does a Chaplain expect from a patient?
- The importance of the trilogy: chaplain, patient and family member
- Write a personal experience based on the information in this chapter

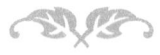

CHAPTER 3
LITERATURE REVIEW

Theological and Psychological Basis for Spiritual Assessments and Current Spiritual Assessment Model

The following instruments were considered: Personal View Survey (PVS), Sense of Coherence Scale (SOC), and Seeking of Noetic Goals (SONG). They are selected for "the measurement of meaning in life" (Young, 2009, p. 5). The same approach is found in the Underwood (1999) study: "The model includes sociocultural, psychological, physical and spiritual aspects of life, around a central integrative core" (para. 1). "The 20-item Seeking of Noetic Goals (SONG) test was developed by Crumbaugh ... and was designated to measure the need/motivation to discover meaning. The term 'Noetic' refers to uniquely human resources, such goals, purposes, creativity, love and humor" (Schulenberg, Baczwaski, & Buchanan, 2013, para. 1) as combined items that will do the assessment more accurately. The ideas described in these models of assessment oriented chaplain to perform these research and develop later an assessment tool that chaplains are using as a guide especially for Palliative Care Patients found in the Daily Census Sheet Report provided to chaplains in the daily basis.

Chaplain Identity

The initiatives of the chaplain will play a great role in the way hospitals develop spiritual backbone in treating patients. In the chaplain's role, in addition to the religious background, these spiritual caregivers should never minimize that their impact on the lives of patients is derived from hospital admission. A good assessment will imply good spiritual treatment, but the way a careless or negligent description of the state of the patient promotes spiritual maltreatment and wrong actions during the process of physical recovery. If a team of chaplains is working, all the spiritual assessment reports of the chaplains who visit a particular patient must generally coincide, even if not totally. For example, it would require teamwork to understand why a Protestant chaplain assessed a Roman Catholic patient as being encouraged and stable, while the priest reported that the same patient showed signs of depression and discouragement. The care and honesty developed during the first visitation must be recognized as huge in the life of the patient. The Spiritual Care Department must take action to fix any disparity when, among the team chaplains, there are so many disparate conclusions. We need to remember to put emphasis especially on the Palliative Care Patients that, in all hospitals, are the main focus of the program. Professional chaplains must offer a knowledgeable hospital patient record.

Stressors in Hospital Patients

One step inside the hospital will make an indelible mark on the patient's life. This mean that the admitted patient expects to be another person by the time he/she is discharged. "A 2012 study from Neurology suggested that in elderly patients, cognitive declines more than double after a hospital stay, affecting patients' thinking and memory skills. The longer the hospitalization, the greater the effect" (Cemental, 2019, para. 1). Changes will occur in their behavior, spiritual views, description of society's role, family relationships, and definitely, in their relationship with the chaplains. Some of them will openly express hatred of the name of God; others will show deep reverence for His holy name. Some post-surgery patients will pour out an attitude of isolation and/or independence. They will reject family involvement in their post-surgery recovery process. Others will grow to be more family-oriented, expecting that a family member be in the patient's room day and night. We also observed a very demanding attitude toward the medical team and expressions of discontent and criticism in spite of the quality attention from the medical team. Depression is also very common after surgery. Patients may seemingly become questioning, demanding immediate responses about how to prepare to go heaven since they feel that their day is coming. Chaplains must be prepared to give an accurate response, but also speak carefully because many patients need responses that engage with their viewpoint of the world, but not the viewpoint of the chaplain.

The concept of palliative care patients varies from one health center to another, but the original concept still remains. Patients' spiritual needs must be addressed and the requirement to find quality and appropriate care are in the hands of the chaplains. The Roswell Park Comprehensive Cancer Center protocol follows what the Joint Commission defines as

> integrating effective communication, cultural competence, and patient and family-centered care into the care delivery system at the end of life. Addressing the patient's communication needs is essential, and in some cases, the hospital may need to meet the communication needs of the patient's surrogate decision maker or family members to involve them in care planning and discussions. (Wilson-Stronks, Schyve, Cordero, Rodríguez, & Youdelman, 2010, p. 33)

There is a very careful assessment and reassessment until the final decision is made.

When the patient is ready, the whole team has the responsibility of informing the patient of the situation, but as well as the possible steps that may be taken.

> The goal of palliative care is to prevent and relieve suffering and to support the best possible quality of life for patients and their families, regardless of the stage of the disease or the need for other therapies. Palliative care is both a philosophy of care and an organized, highly structured system for delivering care.
>
> Palliative care expands traditional disease-model medical treatments to include the goals of enhancing quality of life for patient and family, optimizing function, helping with decision-making and providing opportunities for personal growth. As such, it can be delivered concurrently with life-prolonging care or as the main focus of care. Palliative care is operationalized through effective management of pain and other distressing symptoms, while incorporating psychosocial and spiritual care according to patient/family needs, values, beliefs and culture(s). (Gunten, 2020, paras. 1-2)

During my activities inside the hospital, it is very common to find people who are not aware of the patients' responsibilities and privileges. Many reasons can bring about this situation. The patients may just want to be healed and go home. Sometimes, the family is completely ignorant of how the palliative care team is trying to work, and then there is an opportunity to engage with them by presenting the issues clearly in order to avoid misinterpretation regarding treatment and adding more uncertainty to the life of patient.

> The WHO's definition of palliative care stresses improving not only the quality of life of patients facing incurable diseases but also their families by providing relief from the pain and suffering that includes the psychosocial and spiritual needs as well. (Sharma et al., 2013, para. 1)
>
> A study by Schultz, Lulav-Grinwald, and Bar-sela (2014) is very relevant concerning the importance of spiritual care in patients with cancer: "Data from 364 oncology patient questionnaires found 41% interest in spiritual care, as compared to 35%-54% in American studies. Having previously been visited by a spiritual caregiver predicted patient interest in further spiritual care" (para. 3).

As we can see, the role of the chaplain in close coordination with the medical team is vital. Having both work in harmony with the same goal for the care of the patients and their families will bring the peace and support that every palliative care patient deserves. In the stressful situation that surrounds the close members of the family and friends, the medical team and chaplain always need to remember that "patients with serious, potentially life-threatening illness and their families are very vulnerable and may be initially frightened about the prospect of receiving palliative care" (Quill & Miller, 2014, p. 50). This initiative that was initially planned emphasized and concerned the adult population, but is now projected for the child population.

The International Children's Palliative Care Network (ICPCN) that was celebrated in February 2014 and previously in South Korea in 2005 coincided with the statement of the WHO:

Palliative care for children represents a special, albeit closely related field to adult palliative care and is the active total care of the child's body, mind and spirit, and also involves giving support to the family. It begins when illness is diagnosed, and continues regardless of whether or not a child receives treatment directed at the disease. Health providers must evaluate and alleviate a child's physical, psychological, and social distress. Effective palliative care requires a broad multidisciplinary approach that includes the family and makes use of available community resources; it can be successfully implemented even if resources are limited. It can be provided in tertiary care facilities, in community health centres and even in children's homes. (Downing et al., 2013, para. 3)

Gramling and Gramling (2019) also added,

Palliative care means patient and family-centered care that optimizes quality of life by anticipating, preventing, and treating suffering. So, this is the National Consensus Project definition that's been adopted by Medicare, and I think that you're going to see it in multiple places. But what is unique to this definition is that last word: suffering. In the context of medical education there are few disciplines that have the honor of being focused on this concept of suffering as opposed to disease. (para. 1)

The dual philosophies that led the medical and psychological assessments for centuries is becoming more and more obsolete.

Evidence-based Spiritual Interventions

Amazing statistics is found, 55 to 65 % of Americans that religion is important, wellbeing relationship also has been proved, this research tried to see the influence of the religion in the various facets of the human life. Like Edmonds point out in his book "in the Christian beliefs that the value of any person commences in the grace of Christ: a graceful life" (Edmonds, 2011, p. 372). Relationship between Religion and spirituality in reference of the physical or mental health is based on cross-sectional (results but not causes) findings.

> Approximately 80% of research on R/S and health involves studies on mental health. One would expect stronger relationships between R/S and mental health since R/S involvement consists of psychological, social, and behavioral aspects that are more "proximally" related to mental health than to physical health. In fact, we would not expect any direct or immediate effects of R/S on physical health, other than indirectly through intermediary psychosocial and behavioral pathways. (Koenig, 2011, page. 34).

Another big issue is about positive emotions: "Positive emotions include well-being, happiness, hope, optimism, meaning and purpose, high self-esteem, and a sense of control over life. Related to positive emotions are positive psychological traits such as altruism, being kind or compassionate, forgiving, and grateful." (Koenig, 2011 page 34).

Health professionals in all settings should take a lesson from their patients.

> National guidelines in the United States recommend that spiritual assessment be included with most or

all patients. However, surveys show that over 95% of patients say that no health professional has ever inquired about their spiritual or religious beliefs. Furthermore, most health professionals indicate that they have never been taught how or why to incorporate spiritual or religious assessment into their patient history (Larimore, 2017, para. 1).

A growing consensus exists regarding the importance of spiritual assessment. For instance, the largest health care accrediting body in the United States, the Joint Commission on Accreditation of Healthcare Organizations (JCAHO), now requires the administration of a spiritual assessment. Although most practitioners endorse the concept of spiritual assessment, studies suggest that social workers have received little training in spiritual assessment. To address this gap, the current article reviews the JCAHO requirements for conducting a spiritual assessment and provides practitioners with guidelines for its proper implementation. In addition to helping equip practitioners in JCAHO- accredited settings who may be required to perform such an assessment, the spiritual assessment template profiled in this article may also be of use to practitioners in other settings. (Hodge, 2006, para. 1)

The research method used in this project was qualitative. Quantitative is a method of research that relies on measuring variables using a numerical system, analyzing these measurements using any of a variety of statistical models, and reporting relationships and associations among the studied variables. For example, these variables may be test scores for measurements of reaction time. The goal of gathering this quantitative data is to understand, describe, and predict the nature of a phenomenon, particularly through the development of models and theories (Alfieri,

2015, para. 1). Quantitative research techniques include experiments and surveys. This method was not used in the present research.

The best measurement of R/S is the ten-item Intrinsic Religiosity instrument developed by Hoe. The shortest measure is the Duke Religion Index, while the most comprehensive is the Fetzer Institute Brief Multidimensional Measure of Religiousness/Spirituality; combining measurement tools is acceptable. When analyzing data, the correct procedure is always to follow an analysis plan, technically known as a statistical analysis plan, where variables to be measured are also explained (for example, an ordinary variable might be test grades from A to F. The website for these measurements is free of charge for statistical calculations, but a statistician is needed for grants and publications. Positive psychological traits related to health behaviors, positive emotions, and so on are explanatory variables that may be causally related to both R/S and physiological functions. Genetic, environmental, and epigenetic factors can also alter the relationship of R/S The effects of using scales to determine the influence of R/S using predictors and outcomes in different aspects of the life are an enormous part of the presentation of the paper, as are matters of publication and writing grant requests which also need to be included (Koenig, 2011, p. 253).

Spiritual and Psychological Research

Psycho-oncology: Reason/Results

The medical definition of psycho-oncology is as follows:

> Psycho-oncology addresses the two major psychological dimensions of cancer: (1) the psychological responses of patients to cancer at all stages of the disease, and that of their families and caretakers; and (2) the psychological, behavioral and social factors that may influence the disease process"(Shiel, 2018, para. 1).

Watson (2019) said:

> Psycho-Oncology is concerned with the psychological, social, behavioral, and ethical aspects of cancer. This subspecialty addresses the two major psychological dimensions of cancer: the psychological responses of patients to cancer at all stages of the disease, and that of their families and caretakers; and the psychological, behavioral and social factors that may influence the disease process. Psycho-oncology is an area of multi-disciplinary interest and has boundaries with the major specialties in oncology: the clinical disciplines (surgery, medicine, pediatrics, radiotherapy), epidemiology, immunology, endocrinology, biology, pathology, bioethics, palliative care, rehabilitation medicine, clinical trials research and decision making, as well as psychiatry and psychology. (para. 1)

Social Worker/Pastoral Care Personnel and Palliative Care Patients

Chaplains work very closely with social workers as a team. Chaplains have the opportunity of getting relevant information during patient visits that other members of the medical team may not because time limitations are not a problem for most chaplains. Today's studies promote the open relationship of chaplains with other medical branches (Peteet & D'Ambra, 2011, para. 1). As an example, during my first visit with a palliative care patient, he mentioned that he would like to spend more time in the hospital. Most patients are usually eager to be discharged quickly, but this was not the case with this particular patient because he was homeless. In another case, a young, terminally ill mother with three little children was crying. When the chaplain asked why she was weeping, she did not even mention her concern about her own impending death; her major concern was who was going to take care of the children since their father never showed any interest in them. Good relationships with the Social Work Department is so important when we care for a patient.

Bauer (2014) said:

> Working together is a real gain for the patient. Chaplains refer to a social worker and psycho oncologists at the same these professionals refer the patient to the spiritual care provider. Oncology social workers provide information on resources, medical and insurance coverage, and how to talk to your family and the children in your lives about cancer. We are patient and family advocates. We provide assistance in coping with the diagnosis to patients and families all along the disease continuum, teach relaxation techniques to reduce anxiety, lead psycho-educational support groups, help individuals transition to survivorship, and conduct research about all of the above! We also provide support to our colleagues around burnout and compassion fatigue to help them manage the stressors and loss associated with working in oncology. (para. 3)

Code of Ethics Implications for a
Spiritual Care Assessment

Most of the Roswell Park hospital has a detailed code of ethics specifically for chaplains that every new chaplain hired into Spiritual Care must sign as a demonstration of agreement.

> The development of DSM, from its fourth edition, brought a change into the approach towards

religion and spirituality in the context of clinical diagnosis. Introducing V-code 62.89 has increased the possibility of differential diagnosis between religion/ spirituality and health/psychopathology. The emphasis on manifestation of cultural diversity has enabled non-reductive and non-pathologising insight into the problems of religious and spirituality. (Prusak, 2016, p. 175)

In general, the code of ethics that is mandatory for all care professionals is also applied to chaplains:

Enhancing human development throughout the lifespan; honoring diversity and embracing a multicultural approach in support of the worth, dignity, potential, and uniqueness of people within their social and cultural contexts; promoting social justice; safeguarding the integrity of the counselor–client relationship; and practicing in a competent and ethical manner. These professional values provide a conceptual basis for the ethical principles enumerated below. These principles are the foundation for ethical behavior and decision making. The fundamental principles of professional ethical behavior are autonomy, or fostering the right to control the direction of one's life; nonmaleficence, or avoiding actions that cause harm; beneficence, or working for the good of the individual and society by promoting mental health and well-being; justice, or treating individuals equitably and fostering fairness and equality; fidelity, or honoring commitments and keeping promises, including fulfilling one's responsibilities of trust in professional relationships; and veracity, or dealing truthfully with individuals with whom counselors come into professional contact. (ACA, 2014, p. 24)

The code of ethics that was discussed earlier needs to be revised and studied at least once a year. At Roswell, this is a mandatory review for all employees. The care of the patient and his or her safety is a great priority. The code of ethics could be summarized as the four main core issues that need to be remembered during any contact with patients:

Moral principles of respect for autonomy (the obligation to respect the decision making capacities of autonomous persons); non-maleficence (the obligation to avoid causing harm); beneficence (obligations to provide benefits and to balance benefits against risks); and justice (obligations of fairness in the distribution of benefits and risks). (Beauchamp & Childress, 2012, para. 2)

HIPAA Regulations/Chaplain in Complaint

The HIPAA security rule requires healthcare practitioners and professionals to secure PHI (protected health information) from data breaches, deletions, and other problems. The law's requirements are demanding and can be hard to understand, but I will do my best to make it easy.

To start, there are three areas of HIPAA compliance:

- Administrative measures to ensure patient data is correct and accessible to authorized parties.
- Physical measures to prevent physical theft and loss of devices containing electronic PHI.
- Technical technology-related measures to protect networks and devices from data breaches and unauthorized access.

These three components represent nearly every supporting aspect of one's business: policies, record keeping, technology, and building safety. In this sense, HIPAA requires that all employees be on the same page and working together to protect patient data.

A look at each of these areas will show what is needed to achieve HIPAA compliance. (Alliedhealth, 2019, paras. 5-7)

Roswell Park Comprehensive Cancer Center Pastoral Care Policy

The spiritual care policy applied at Roswell is no different than that of many hospitals in the United States and around the world. Patient care goes far beyond just physical care. An individual having treatment and facing the uncertainty of life and death has serious questions that seek answers. This is the place where spiritual care centers into action. Whatever may have been the previous health conditions of the patient, for the first time the fragility of the life is understood in its real dimension. Patients are looking for answers and see in the spiritual care provider relief for their thirsty souls. Rodgers (2013) said,

> Among the basic spiritual needs that might be addressed within the normal daily activity of healthcare include: - the need to be listened to - the need to give and receive unconditional love - the need to be understood - the need to be valued as a human being - the need for forgiveness, hope and trust - the need to explore beliefs and values - the need to express feelings honestly - the need to find meaning and purpose in life. (p. 3)

What an important task the chaplain can deliver every time he/she enters in contact with patient. There is no place to take an intervention in the life of a patient that is uncaring or that may be hurtful. Every minute has to be extremely valued and used to benefit the suffering. This is the reason Rodgers summarized the work and policy of the hospital as being to identify and assess the level of need for spiritual, pastoral and religious care. • support staff as they provide spiritual care to patients, their relatives and careers, both in hospital and in community settings. • participate in training programs for clinical and non-clinical staff and students, and in staff induction. • And religious care as part of the multidisciplinary team by visiting, listening to and supporting patients, their relatives and careers, and staff. • offer religious ministries and acts of worship at the bedside or other appropriate places. (p. 3)

The list could continue as the hospital tries to serve those who come looking for care in the best way possible.

- Roswell Park follows the same rules that are applied to most research centers. Every new chaplain must read it in order to comply with the regulations established by the board of directors that directs the life of the hospital.
- Spiritual Care Assessment. In this area, most chaplains use what was updated four years ago. Lay chaplains use a hard copy, but professional chaplains use sensor sheets in order to take notes during the assessment and later consolidate the information into daily electronic charting following the format established by the hospital and in accordance with HIPAA regulations and the JCAHO.

Spiritual Care in Hospitals

There is abundant literature in this area. I truly believe that spiritual and psychological care must go together for the good of the patient. The Pennsylvania health group, for example, serves 2.6 million patients and has experienced its own benefits of putting a huge effort in place that combines the psychological aspect together with the medical:

> Three years ago, the facility was one of the three pediatric community centers selected to pilot an integrated-care program in which primary care physicians, psychologists, nurses and other medical professionals work together to diagnose and treat physical and psychological health problems. Gianfagna and other physicians learned how to screen for depression, anxiety, attention deficit hyperactivity disorder and several other mental health conditions, and now have a full-time psychologist and several psychology residents down the hall available for one-on-one and group therapy or for consultations on a variety of mental and behavioral health conditions. (Novotney, 2014, p. 46)

Others are more focused on spiritual care such as the Spirituality and the Spiritual Rating Scale (McSherry, Draper, & Kendrick, 2002, p. 723), and the results are very strongly based on evidence.

This kind of practice is being expanded across the country with amazing results. Most centers conclude that it is not possible to separate the psyche from the soma, the soul from the body. Both are integrated and relate to one another. The concept of dualism introduced by Plato is becoming more and more obsolete, at least for now, in the medical arena. "Research clearly shows that psychological, behavioral and social factors are key drivers of health problems seen in primary-care settings" (Novotney, 2014, p. 46). Positive results when addressing these issues are demonstrated in the quality of life of the terminally ill patient, but "the current emphasis on patient 'choice' in government strategies is meaningless without an infrastructure within which choices can realistically be met, and can add to the pressure on doctors, patients and families" (Brannan et al., 2016, p. 13).

Unfortunately, not everyone will be able to fulfill that desire. On numerous occasions, I got someone's request at the last minute. For medical and internal hospital policies, the patient has to stay in hospital until life is gone. Often misunderstanding the role of palliative care in the life of the patient makes life more difficult for families and also gives the medical team more stress. For example, we very often see discrepancies over the future of the patient during family meetings at the hospital. This kind of situation arises when influenced by psychological burn-out or religious orientation that was not addressed in previous meetings. For example, one may take the case of a husband requesting hundreds of prayers around the world, believing that the will of God is to wait until his wife stops breathing. But she is already breathing artificially and was declared brain dead one week ago. Untrained clergy easily nurture this kind of assumptions that has no biblical or medical support. This, in turn, creates a problem for the medical team and psychological burnout for the families taking care of the patient. The same situation has been observed in a wife who promised her husband she would never leave him while he was in the hospital. At the beginning, it seemed interesting, and the ICU administrators did not prevent it until it escalated into chaos, moving the Ethics Committee of the hospital to make the difficult decision of removing the wife from the ICU room after 25 days of staying inside the room because of her promise.

Spiritual and psychological issues need to be taken seriously when patient is admitted. Otherwise, there could be devastating consequences that shake the foundation of the most prominent hospital. Chaplains must show that "the loveliness of the character of Christ will be seen in His fallowers. It was His delight to do the will of God" (White, 1988, p. 151). The Israeli study presented in the Biomedical Med Central, for example, states that "spiritual care addressed a key patient need{1, 2}in a manner that has significant benefits, such as improved quality of life{1, 3, 4},well-being{5}, and reduced anxiety, despair, or depression,{6, 8}that have been demonstrated cross –culturally{9}. Spiritual care has become an integral part of palliative care {10.11} and should be seen as an element of providing care for the whole person {12}" (Schultz et al., 2014, p. 14).

Good assessment will provide a good goal and then a good plan for the patient.

> In the context of illness and suffering, quality of life is a multidimensional, dynamic, and subjective perspective of health-related satisfaction. Research shows that this health-related satisfaction is connected to spiritual and religious well-being. (Stoltzfus, 2013, p. 119)

In general, persons who have been interned as palliative care patients seemed to want to exercise every tool possible in the recovery process or to prepare for departure. The important clue in this process is discovering the level of religiosity or spirituality that will give the chaplain the spiritual roadmap for the next few days in order to engage first with the patient, but also to reach the confidence of the family and other community systems that influence patient behavior.

I myself have found it very important to define the terms being used with the patients themselves. Many Roman Catholic patients believe that the presence of the chaplain at the bedside is a sign that the end is near for them and in some cases, a threat that needs to be avoided. The same attitude is seen when trying to introduce palliative care to patients with serious and potentially life-threatening illnesses. They feel frightened and confused until they realize the great benefit offered to them in the plan. Therefore "palliative medicine seeks to provide the best quality of life for patients and families using a model in which the goals of care are collaboratively developed with care providers according to wishes of patients and families" (Issues in Palliative Care, 2013, para. 2).

Others have spiritual perspectives, especially at the present time.

> A growing contingent of Americans—particularly young Americans—identify as "spiritual but not religious." Masthead member Joy wanted to understand why. On our call with Emma Green, The Atlantic's religion writer, Joy asked, "What are they looking for?" Because the term "spiritual" can be interpreted in so many different ways, it's a tough question to answer. (Kitchener, 2018)

I have talked to people who spent a lot of time reflecting on this question and I came away with some helpful observations which may be important in the context of the major shift happening in American faith. This may help to define the chaplain as a perfect support during the journey of recovery. That is the reason for solid spiritual screening and rescreening aimed to cover the real needs of the patient, but also the personal effectiveness of the spiritual care provider.

As I mentioned earlier, if we work as a team, the effectiveness at the time of life transition of the palliative care patient will be outstanding. Most hospitals are taking this position, but others are still reluctant to assume this kind of position. According to Novotney (2014), a researcher at the Pennsylvania health group that put this approach of 100% collaboration between medical and psychological teams into practice, "anecdotal reports show that our physicians are feeling less stressed and more prepared because they have the screening instruments they need and our guidance" (p. 46). In my setting, the relationship includes social workers who display great ability when visiting patients, but at the same time, engagement with the pastoral care team. Studies have found that social workers' interest is centered in solving problems that affect health and contribute the greatest benefit for the greatest number of people.

This commitment requires work from an interdisciplinary group. Nothing important is possible by trying to work alone. All sectors must embrace a cooperative effort with one unique goal—the wellness of the one who is suffering. Social workers and the pastoral care team have one thing in common at Roswell Park Comprehensive Cancer Center: listening to the patient. While most of the medical personnel do not have enough time to dedicate to each patient, the palliative care team is there to sit down, engage with the patient's emotional and spiritual burdens and seek to supply those spiritual or psychological needs. Most patients are thirsting for someone to listen to them, not just someone who sits down to review the physical development and procedures that usually raise more questions than responses. Sometimes just sitting down by the bed of the patient says much more than a hundred words. A Taoist tale of the woodcarver gives us an idea of what this means. "Sometimes silence does what words cannot." As visitors, we need to make encounter authentic so that those few moments together with the patient may shape both lives in that moment and beyond. The main concern when visiting for the first time is the way you present yourself to them. Those few seconds will determine whether the moment will be a time of welcome or rejection. The real encounter with them requires work, dedication and patience. Every professional chaplain and member of the psychological discipline must recognize that in every bed of the hospital there is a human being who is afraid, vulnerable, and worried.

Working in this capacity in a hospital invites a profound meditation, incessant multi-tasking, and little time to pause or reflect. This is the main reason why the chaplain or the social worker must think seriously when he has the list of patients in his hand: Who is this person I am going to visit? The real tendency in modern society is to see things as numbers. Bank account numbers, driver's license numbers, student ID numbers, and so on. The Palliative Care team receives the bed or room numbers of the patient to be visited during the day. The number setting is there, but chaplains and social workers must avoid the temptation of seeing bed or room number. There is a person; a unique person in the universe whose handling of his life may be for the last time. We need to enter into the real life of the patient, his personal history, his life before he heard a stage-4 cancer diagnosis, or doctors saying to her you have to go home because there is no more treatment available to you, everything is over. Is necessary now to interact with the whole person together with his strengths and vulnerabilities, with ideas rooted in beliefs, tradition, and culture. Some of them are deep in Epicureanism whose concept of death is far away of the chaplain's concept of preparation. One of them might think "that death is not harm to the person who dies and those persons can neither be harmed nor wronged by events that occur after their deaths" (Taylor, 2013, para. 1). The unique world that we bring needs to understood as special when the painful transition is knocking at our doors.

I believe that chaplains and social workers fight with their own egos most of the time. The competing persona (ego) often gets transferred into one's manner of relating/communicating with patients. One's personal agenda is as dangerous as dynamite in the hands of the novice. We need to hear what the patient hears; learning to walk in the patient's shoes must be our goal. Offering inappropriate care to the individual can be more hurtful than offering no help at all. There is the possibility of praying for the family of the person when they did not request it and have no interest in that request. We need to focus on the patient and know well who they are and what they care about. The professional competence and ability to listen and observe what the patient is saying to you is at play here. The mind of the chaplain must be focused on only the need of the patient at the precise moment of the intervention.

Roswell Park Comprehensive Cancer Center's philosophy in patient visitation is based on "quality more than quantity." The patient's time with the chaplain is sacred and deserves such respect and quality as to be accountable to the hospital administration, but also to God. The Bible clearly states in Matt 25:40, 45, "In as much as you did not do it to one of these least of these, you did not do it to me."

> We believe that all the dimensions of our beings carry the potential to do good. We celebrate the gifts of being human: our intelligence and capacity for observation and reason, our senses and ability to appreciate beauty, our creativity, our feelings and emotions. We cherish our bodies as well as our souls. We can use our gifts to offer love, to work for justice, to heal injury, to create pleasure for ourselves and others. . . .
>
> "Just to be is a blessing. Just to live is holy," the great twentieth-century Rabbi Abraham Heschel wrote. Unitarian Universalists affirm the inherent worth and dignity of each person as a given of faith—an unshakeable conviction calling us to self-respect and respect for others. (Parker, 2019, p. 4)

The value of people is immense, and we need to see them in that perspective.

Ethics and Spiritual Care Assessment

From the moment the patient steps into the hospital, different departments are ready to utilize the best assessment possible to establish the goals and medical plan for the individual. Similarities exist when counselors make assessments in the mental health area. "Researchers can generate the potential for benefit to all stakeholders within the research process through maintaining a wide understanding of ethical and emotionally intelligent behaviors" (Hurley, Linsley, & MacLeod, 2012, p. 455). The spiritual care department does the same thing, and we add something extra that we call the "re-assessment" process. All these activities have an important purpose, to establish the roadmap toward physical, emotional, and intellectual restoration. All assessment has intrinsic responsibilities that start with the health care provider, the kind of assessment tool that he will utilize, and is the one who goes to the patient who is ready and willing to enter into the assessment process.

There is not just one actor in any assessment. Both will play a big role of responsibility. Thinking about in the assessment giver for example that must be a representative of the hospital and well prepared, with the credentials and training to corroborate this delicate endeavor but also with the capability to emerge patient disposition to engage in an honest and fruitful moment of assessment. I found that two traditions of medical ethics are used in the United States, deontological and teleological...they opposed each other on most issues. From deontological ethics (duty ethics) of abstract, universal, rational rules of moral obligations, ethics is a crucial branch in medicine guiding good medical practice. It deals with the moral dilemmas arising due to conflicts in duties/obligations and the faced consequences. They are based on four fundamental principles, i.e., autonomy, beneficence, nonmaleficence, and justice. Much of modern medical ethics deals with the moral dilemmas arising in the context of patient's autonomy and the fundamental principles of informed consent and confidentiality. Ethics deals with choices, decisions/actions based on the choice and the duties and obligations of a doctor to the best interest of the patient.

> Medical ethics is a sensible branch of moral philosophy and deals with conflicts in obligations/ duties and their potential outcome. Two strands of thought exist in ethics regarding decision-making: deontological and utilitarian. In deontological approach, outcomes/consequences may not just justify the means to achieve it while in utilitarian approach; outcomes determine the means and

greatest benefit expected for the greatest number. In brief, deontology is patient-centered, whereas utilitarianism is society-centered. Although these approaches contradict each other, each of them has their own substantiating advantages and disadvantages in medical practice. Over years, a trend has been observed from deontological practice to utilitarian approach leading to frustration and discontentment. Health care systems and practitioners need to balance both these ethical arms to bring congruity in medical practice. (Mandal, Ponnambath, & Parija, 2016, para. 1)

In Roswell Park Comprehensive Cancer Center, both traditions are important, although most of the chaplains tend to use more deontological assessments when trying to bridge the chaplains' personal responsibility, using their own ethical-cultural background and also their "vicarious condition" in the sight of the organizations that supports the ministry (Pastoral Care Department). Roswell Park Comprehensive Cancer Center has its own code of ethics that must be read by new hires/volunteers in hospital affairs prior to engaging in patient visitation. Christian chaplains on the one hand will try to put all their knowledge of traditions or Biblical concepts into this kind of assessment tool; Jewish chaplains will emphasize the use of the Law, the Prophets and Writings to engage worried, hospitalized Jewish members (the book of Psalms is preferred); Indian chaplains will emphasize other spiritual factors during their assessment and interventions; Muslim chaplains who are not always an Imam must provide support using existential tools to help their community; and so on. The influence of one's own cultural background is so great that it can affect important decision like "Do not resuscitate" (DNR). We are not in a position to judge them or try to say which one is correct or not. The person who is lying on the bed is unique and has had unique and particular experiences. We always need to remember their individual freedoms and the right to refuse anything, and that includes medical treatments. We need also remember that patients entering the hospital have their own programmed psyche that is basically composed of integrated systems and learned behaviors that make the process of health care assessment very intense at a particular moment. This is why chaplains must at least be trained in an informal assessment.

> Informal spiritual assessment may be accomplished at any time during the medical encounter. . . .
>
> Because most patients use symbolic and metaphoric language when expressing spiritual thoughts, spiritual assessment often involves listening carefully to the stories that patients tell regarding their lives and illness and then interpreting the spiritual issues involved. (Anandarajah & Hight, 2001, pp. 30, 33)

No one can change what they learned from childhood and practiced all their lives in a matter of a couple of days or months. Atheists' behaviors are different to the believer's counterparts. I remember, for example, the case of a well-known writer who was grieving process whom I was assigned to visit. I never was a successful visitor with her because she refused to see a chaplain. She was an atheist and had the right to do that during her last days of life. On other hand, another chaplain had an agnostic patient who refused any pastoral visitants, but his wife was a devout Wesleyan. We are not in the hospital to change the philosophies of the patients, but we are there to serve in the best way possible. When the agnostic husband passed away, his wife called the Protestant chaplain to preside over his religious funeral; this was accepted as a part of the grieving process of the wife and family. Chaplains use tools like assessment in order to walk in the shoes of the patients; they will use every means possible to see through the lenses of the patient.

The human mind and soul are the gateway to the life of a person. The condition of these two are often related to the life one leads, and it is safe to say that one who is pure in mind and soul is the enlightened one. With a fast-paced lifestyle, and a wide range of technological products, the mind and soul has certainly been corrupted to a large degree. (Chowdhury, 2016, para. 1)

There are important reasons that bringing one's own agenda either during assessment or during visitation or using the moment of pain and anxiety to proselytize, will be disastrous and unethical. These are very important topics that I learned during CPE at Sisters of Charities Hospital a short time ago. However, above all, the first concern of healthcare ethics should be the person who is seeking health care, rather than the professionals or institutions that provide it. Medical ethics is a sensible branch of moral philosophy and deals with conflicts in obligations/duties and their potential outcome. Two strands of thought exist in ethics regarding decision-making: deontological and utilitarian.

In the deontological approach, outcomes/ consequences may not justify the means to achieve it, while in the utilitarian approach, outcomes may determine the means and greatest benefit expected for the greatest number. In brief, deontology is patient-centered, whereas utilitarianism is society-centered. Although these approaches contradict each other, each of them has its own substantiating advantages and disadvantages in medical practice. (Mandal, Ponnambath, & Parija, 2016, pp. 6-7)

This is what I believe: Many patients, for example, do not have a Health Care Proxy because they do not understand its function;

others do not care as a way of avoiding the present reality (which is very common especially with recently diagnosed patients). Careless health care providers will explain (the "mopping process") until the patient sees the urgent need of providing a trustworthy person's name to act in his/her behalf. Fortunately, the individual's culture is not static, but prone to change or assimilate new ways of living/skills/knowledge that will affect his/her entire life from that time on. The wish of the patient, his/her culture, and the setting must be taken into account.

> One would think that with all the emphasis on patient autonomy and advance care planning (ACP) that patients' wishes would be respected. The Study to Understand Prognoses and Preferences for Outcomes and Risks of Treatments (SUPPORT)—which involved over 9,000 patients—sadly dispelled this optimistic belief. The first phase of the study was observational and took place over two years in five major teaching hospitals. It found that nearly half of physicians did not know that their patient did not want CPR, and a similar percentage of DNR orders were written within two days of death. Over a third of study subjects who died spent ten or more days in the intensive care unit, and half of conscious patients reported moderate or severe pain more than half the time in the days leading up to their deaths. (Macauley, 2018, p. 26)

Chaplains play an active role in this process. Correspondence and coordination with the Palliative Care Department is important and necessary. At Roswell Park Comprehensive Cancer Center, coordination with the director of Palliative Care Unit is expected early every morning after having the list of palliative care patients in hand.

Effectiveness of Current Spiritual Care Assessment Models

We are going to analyze the impact in the life of every palliative care patient. There are many that offer the best, but much of the model's effectiveness will be seen in adapting to hospital culture and needs. Roswell Park Comprehensive Cancer Center, for example, has the great influence of the Puchalski FICA model that contains four basic questions that need responses: Faith or Beliefs, Importance and Influence, Community, and Address. Specific open-ended questions are shared in order to get the most accurate and also that the patient has the right to respond or not. Freedom of religion (Bill of Rights) clearly establishes that people can have a religion or not, but the chaplains' question will clarify it. For example: Do you consider yourself spiritual/religious? This gives the patient the opportunity to reflect on his own stay. Lying down in a bed for hours and days drives an individual to an honest response. Most of them are seeking strength from their own spiritual assets (praying, repeating the Rosary, condemning others, etc.); others are learning how to use them. When the patient starts being more open and the chaplain uses the right tone of voice and is seated (standing up is the worst posture for interviewing a patient), we can ask whether their beliefs have influenced their behavior during that illness. The response or lack of response will lead the chaplain to the next step in the intervention. Careful observations (not just listening to the responses), observing body language, level of mental stress, and capacity to interact are the basics tools when intervention is needed. Doctors are very careful when questioning patients to determine factors that will lead to physical interventions (labs, tests, surgeries); chaplain intervention leads to discovering the early signs of spiritual worsening in order to apply the proper spiritual medication or procedure. Beth Lenegan and the Pastoral Care team have adapted FICA's model and as a result, have their own way of making reassessment procedures. However, any assessment must follow a selected strategy of assessment. "The three major strategies are interviewing, observing behavior, and psychological testing" (Groth-Marnat, 2009, p. 67). Chaplains are prepared and competent to follow these kinds of protocols. The Joint Commission (2011), when delineating elements of performances enlist the patients' religion and spiritual beliefs, values and preferences the following:

- living situation
- leisure and recreation activities
- military service history
- peer group
- social factors
- ethnic and cultural factors
- financial status
- vocational or educational background
- legal history and communication skills.

Having the privilege of being with a patient is a wonderful opportunity to enter in their realms, to discover what they truly need. The reliability and validity of an assessment will determine the grade of the outcomes. According to Borneman (2018) who presented a preliminary clinical evaluation of FICA's, they used n=76 and a mean age of 57 as a pattern of evaluation by using open ended questions to rate the importance of faith belief in their life on a 0 (not important) to 5(very important) scale. The mean score of 8.40 indicated that spirituality was important to patients, and data confirmed that the FICA was effective for assessing several dimensions of spirituality based on correlation with spirituality indicators in the Quality of Life tool-spiritual domain. (para. 4)

I found that other hospitals use different models such as the Hope Assessment:

H–sources of hope, strength, comfort, meaning, peace, love and connection

O–the role of organized religion for the patient
P–personal spirituality and practices
E–effects on medical care and end-of-life decisions

Another good assessment instrument emphasizes the "four Rs" that stands for Reflect, React, Reason, and Reflection (Kostelnik, Soderman, Whiren, & Rupiper, 2018, p. 314). Questions like why this is happening to me? religion, and we are there to agree with the individual's belief. Kind of relationship either vertical/horizontal or Restoration (from spiritual distress). Other resources of Spiritual Care Assessments are the Holy Spirit Questionnaire (HSQ), Spiritual Assessment Inventory (SAI) and the Spiritual Well -Being Scale (SWBS). I agree with Koenig (as cited in LaRocca-Pitts, 2009) that a good spiritual assessment has five components: "brevity, memorability, appropriateness, patient-centeredness, and credibility" (para. 1). He also mentioned the following as a tool for a good assessment: "The chaplain-developed FACT stands for: F—Faith (and/or Belief); A—Active (and/or Available, Accessible, Applicable); C—Coping (and/or Comfort)/Conflict (and/or Concern); and T—Treatment" (para. 1).

One of the assessments that has been used frequently in different hospital settings in different ways but very close in content is SIMPLE.

Spirituality (S). When visiting a patient, the first thing to consider about chaplain work is to know where her spirituality is. As human beings and free to exercise every kind of spiritual perspective imaginable, we must place ourselves exactly where the spiritual pendulum is in the patient's life. For many patients, their spirituality rests on the notion of God, the Father, the Son, and the Holy Spirit. This means that your spirituality is entrusted to God with the notion of Christianity. Others simply do not have an idea to formulate the idea of God and prefer to be off this radar and prefer to be under the umbrella of agnosticism. Many of them know that there is something great and supernatural, but they prefer not to identify themselves as God. And they are reducers think about it. They have other more important problems. Questions like:

Where does your source of strength rest? Do you have any beliefs? Who helps you in times of distress? Who is your main support as you walk on this journey? Are you an active member of your religious community? Did you receive the rite of the Anointing of the Sick?

Information (I). Most patients have a lot of personal information that they would like to share with you as a chaplain. This type of narrative is appropriate to share with you as a chaplain, because you are a minister of God, a professional in your field and you access the privacy of the patient due to your personal sensitivity. On one occasion, a 63-year-old patient on her end-of-life patient list has just shared with the chaplain that she wants to meet Jesus and that she is ready. But it was her family that couldn't capture her deep desire and the end of her life doesn't bother him. And she took advantage of the chaplain's visit to vent her feelings and emotions. For chaplains trying to better serve the patient, information is vital and necessary. Questions that can help the chaplain are: Do you attend a religious meeting in your community? How often do you get visits from your family and friends? Do you have any current information from your doctor and nurses?

Doctor (M). This is an important area in the hands of the chaplain because it allows him to glimpse the physical suffering of the patient. You are not a doctor, but as part of the group of caregivers who will nurture the spiritual area of the patient, you must be aware of the physical pain of the patient, for example, it is good to know the level of pain of your patient knowing that 0 is not pain. and 10 is the worst pain. Sometimes medical terminology is important when visiting a patient. For example, on the door there may be this sign: NPO or precautionary measures signs, which to enter to see a patient will need gloves, a gown, glasses and a mask. Now living in the era of COVID-19 there are strict rules that you should be aware of before entering a room where you and your neighbors may be in trouble. The questions that may be asked are: How clearly do you know about your medical problem? Do you understand exactly your current situation? Is your doctor answering all your questions? Are you in pain at the moment? Do you fully know the reason for your medications?

Pastoral (P). Pastoral (P). This has to do with the relationship with local clergy, community leader or relative for whom it is the most important support system in the process. Many of the skates will share multiple supports, others possibly only one and rarely, but none impossible. Questions that could be used are: Do you have any support?, Who is closest to you on this journey? Did your church / leader support you?

Le it go (L). this is the area where the patient finds release from his worries, worries, struggles. Many of them have hiding places that professional chaplains need to explore. These scanned and treated areas provide extensive physical and psychological pain relief. The questions that can be used are: Do you have something in mind that does not give you peace? Is your family fully involved in supporting you? How long did you get a call from your partner? May I invite the priest to visit you? Can I sing / play your favorite song / hymn?

Education (E). This area of assessment will show the chaplain the patient's literacy regarding her own illness and other areas of her life. The questions that can be used are? Is the Bible Important to You? At what level is your disease now? Are you active in your church? Who is your pastor and if I can call him

SIMPLE Evaluation: FORMAT

Name: ....Floor / Bed Sex Age

Hospital Name
Religious Creed / Philosophy
SPIRITUALITY
Supreme Authority: Rites
Death Concept:

INFORMATION
Religious community:
Relationship with the medical / palliative team assistance
MEDICAL
New/Readmission Date
Relationship to God / Wing / Nature:

Specification of your belief: Special Request
No visit

Source of help:

Social

Diagnosis: Level Designated Representative Palliative Patient (NA / POS / Pre-S) Pain Restrictions

Palliative Care Assessmet: Impact in the Life of Patients with Cancer at Roswell Park Comprehensive Cancer Center
Medical Situation: Medications Advance Directives:
PASTORAL
Value of your religious / philosophical community Visits

Spiritual Experience: Request:
LET IT GO:
Conduct: Confession: Spiritual exercise:
EDUCATION
Resources: Demography:
Intellectual Guide Pastoral Information
Expressions Mental health
Ecclesiastical / Philosophical Experience

Psychological Research Regarding Spiritual Care in Hospitals

In the past, only the medicine would apply to the Biomedical Model and it seemed unnecessary to include other means of addressing both simple and complicated medical situations. Nowadays, however, things are constantly updating, and new discoveries and new treatments, especially in cancer patients, are being investigated. Instead of emphasizing only biomedical models, most hospitals are using biopsychosocial models that convene regular treatment, but also address the mental and psychological aspects of the patient.

Psycho-oncology: Reason/Results

Evidence-based treatment that includes quantitative and qualitative research has recognized the real benefits of including the psycho-oncology awareness. Patients must now be observed in their whole spectrum of life that includes both their own struggles and also those of the ones who are supporting them. We never underestimate issues of spirituality, nor of going to exaggeration, as Meador and Levin (2012) mentioned:

Religion is now promoted as a commodity or goods to be used to improve one's health independent of other considerations. Poor outcomes, seen through this lens, are G thus failures of faith—a terrible burden to place on people already suffering from health challenges. (para. 2)

In recent years, attempting to better understand the nature and type of cancer-related distress encountered by patients has led to a better definition of distress, with accompanying prevalence studies of most frequently encountered problems.

These studies have qualitatively and quantitatively demonstrated that cancer is complex and multifactorial (physical, practical, emotional, and spiritual) affecting the quality of life of patients and their families and that standardized screening for distress may be the most effective and efficient way of understanding the patient and the challenges they encounter from time of diagnosis through treatment, recurrent disease, and palliative care. . . . These findings have importantly highlighted key areas of patient concern where psychosocial interventions can be timely, targeted and evidence based. (Bultz, 2016, pp. 118, 120)

Spiritual Care Assessments

In the process of gathering relevant information during a chaplaincy care conversation (the first part of the spiritual assessment), the chaplain listens for or elicits information related to the various f-categories. When one of them is brought up, say the patient's faith or spiritual practice, the chaplain can explore it further by inquiring about the patient's needs in this area. Thesis the A-part of the FACT algoriethm: Access or Available. Although it may not be as neat or as simple as Access or Available, it seeks to determine the patient's needs and desires in relation to the particular f-category presented. The chaplain also listens to discern if the patient has any Anxiety related to this f-category. (Pitts, 2015, p. 53)

Spiritual assessment has been used at Roswell since the beginning of the Spiritual Care Department in 1990 but has changed in form and use. In 2015, chaplains had to use paper forms with the basic questions, but it was not a requirement to chart the information. Since 2016, charting and using electronic medical records has become mandatory. Now we use patient medical records on a daily basis to record all the spiritual information collected during the spiritual assessment or any other kind of interchange with the patients.

Recent Research/Books

Research in every field is very important. For example, research addressing Hispanic delinquency mentions that "cultural arts programming is effective for alleviating depression, anxiety, and related mental health issues as well as bolstering positive familial relations" (Rapp-Pagliccci, Stewart, Rowe, & Miller, 2011, p. 100).

Videos that Refer to Palliative Care Patients

In reference to videos, there are good ones that I can suggest: "Palliative Care: You Are a Bridge"; "Palliative Care Patients: Regaining a Quality Life"; "Palliative Care from Diagnosis to Death"; and "Know the Difference: Hospice vs. Palliative Care."

Chapter Reflections:

- How would you define the theological and psychological basis for spiritual evaluations?
- In your opinion, what would the patient's current spiritual evaluation model look like?
- How important is the identity of the Chaplain?
- Do you agree with the concept of patients in palliative care?
- Why is very careful evaluation and reevaluation so important in making a final decision?
- The importance of ethical evaluation and spiritual care in the patient.
- Your opinion in relation to the evaluation called SIMPLE.

CHAPTER 4
DESCRIPTION OF THE INITIATIVE

A theological basis for the spiritual assessment was developed. Palliative care assessment has the same foundations as the medical diagnosis. "Spiritual assessment during Treatments...inquire about the patient's and family hopes for the future. Asses the level and quality of support they are receiving, What is concerning you the most at this time...what is the most challenging part of this for you? And "What is helping you day by day "What is the most important to you in life? Are these helpful or not?"(Ferrell, 2006 Pag58:4, 59:1)

The reason for the assessment in both areas is to find the basic cause of the symptoms, and that may take numerous steps to find the real problem. Since creation itself, God planned the world; it did not happen by accident, according to Bible and other resources there was a plan right before o the world foundation. : "Who verily was foreordained before the foundation of the world, but was manifest in these last times for you" (1 Pet 1:20 KJV). Similar to God's work for saving humanity, planning and assessing, carefully and with love, is the chaplain's responsibility. Prophets and prophetesses reflected that pattern in God's work. We can imagine how the prophet Daniel predicted things that still resonate in our days. The prophecy of Dan 8:14, for example, is a good example of assessment and planning that is detailed and executed at the precise time: "And he said to me, 'For 2,300 evenings and mornings; then the holy place will be properly restored'" (NAS). Every step and every event from 538 BCE to 1844 CE was planned accurately. No event or action was left out of the plan, and again, the chaplain's job must follow the example of the Master Planner. The Apostle Paul during his ministry never has demonstrated, the Apostle Paul addressing to the Corinthians, told them "Examine yourselves to see whether you are in the faith; test yourselves. Do you not realize that Christ Jesus is in you—unless, of course, you fail the test? (NIV, 2011) "To examine one's self, spiritually, includes an honest look at whether one is truly a believer in Jesus. Along with that, it calls Christians to examine the details and results of their faith, to see if it's according to the truth. It would involve scrutinizing one's own conduct to see how—or if—they follow through on the will of God for their lives" (Bibleref, 2020). The Gospel according to Mark in the Gospel also write writer also mentioned He said to his disciples, "Why are you so afraid? Do you still have no faith?" (Mark 4:40NIV version) Jesus has demonstrated that his is the master of the assessments, like mentioned he assessed with the disciples the lack of faith, the lack of real commitment to his cause. Being afraid and being converted are things that relate to each other. Its convene with attitude, behavior, feelings and a direct response to a stimuli "The devil is very busy about careless hearers, as the fowls of the air go about the seed that lies above ground. Many continue in a barren, false profession, and go down to hell. Impressions that are not deep, will not last. Many do not mind heart-work, without which religion is nothing. Others are hindered from profiting by the word of God, by abundance of the world. And those who have but little of the world, may yet be ruined by indulging the body. "(Christianity, 2020 paragraph 1) The Apostle John, (Revelation 12: 1-17) also enters in the plan of assessment and this is regarding to the woman and the action of the dragon. Interestingly St John includes in his assessment that includes details like "A woman clothed with the sun" "Her head a crown of twelve stars" then goes to the Dragon that had" seven heads and ten horns". This mean observation, attentiveness, detail oriented, but more "I heard a loud voice in heaven saying" implies careful listening. And that is exactly the Palliative Assessment is about. Other texts that support this are Prov 8:22-29; John 1:1-3; 1 Cor 2:7; and 2 Tim 1:9"

A form summarizing the complete psychological, sociological, and spiritual concerns with clearly defined areas of assessment of the patient and their family was developed (Appendix B). To determine the knowledge base and understanding of Spiritual Care Assessment in Palliative Care Patients at Roswell Park Comprehensive Cancer Center, I used the following process. I formulated a semi-structured technique survey conformed to 4 areas and 34 quota to fulfil questions. Every area was selected according to the need of exploration information that will lead to the questions that will solidify the findings among the Palliative Care population. This type of research is called Qualitive Research that "is primarily exploratory research. It is used to gain an understanding of underlying reasons, opinions, and motivations (DeFranzo, 2011, paragraph 2).

The rationale for this study is based in the deep importance and transcendence that can cause in the quality of life of patients and the understanding between medical approach and the spiritual care. The appropriateness is based in two very important levels that relate to the Palliative Care. On one side, every chaplain need to equip with an accurate tool to determine the course of actions to be performed with the patient. In this process of assessment also is related to the family member that obviously is present to carry out the burden of the beloved ones in treatment. For example "one of the many symptoms experienced by those of End of Life pain is the most common and most feared" (Paice, 2006, page 131). Without a good understanding of assessment process care givers can accentuate the struggles or worsen it. "Understanding these barriers will lead the professionals to better educate and better counsel the patients and their families" (Paice, 2006 page 132). The rationale to select the ones will use the survey was based in the kind of interaction that the chaplain is having currently in the hospital. They have to demonstrate direct interaction with palliative patients. The most important criteria to be part of this survey is to being able to spend selected people to do the survey was primarily trained individually, when they seemed understood widely about the survey, words, medical terminologies, etc. the purpose and the methodology, we proceeds with next step which mean the execution of the survey. Like Presser mentions "A careful pilot test conducted by sensitive interviewers is the most direct way of discovering these problem words" (Presser, 2004). We were very aware of the item response theory (IRT) models and the computer adaptive tests (CAT), where a "respondent is presented a question near the middle of the scale range, and an estimate of his total score is constructed based on his response, When they returned the questionnaires, a single statistical method was applied. Two large regression models in which these characteristics were the independent variables and the MTMM reliability or validity estimates were the dependent variables provide estimates of the effect on the reliability or validity of the question characteristics. New items can be coded (aided by the authors' software) and the prediction equation (also automated) used to estimate their quality (Presser, 2004). "In stablishing the breadth and the depth of the interview, it is important that you are able to stablish trust and rapport and assure confidentiality within the limits of the purpose the individual is being assessed. The better the interviewer is able to build trust, the more likely the information will be reliable" (Neukrug, 2010 page 262) The relevance of this research can be seen in the dynamic between a responsible palliative care assessment and the consequent intervention weighed by the kind of individual plan and constructs supporting the Individual Plan. The procedure to select the people was based in the list of chaplains and volunteers that works at Spiritual Care Department. The Director of the program played a great role to select the correct group.

Three spiritual care directors were interviewed. This part was performed with the Director of Spiritual Care at Roswell Park Comprehensive Cancer Center, Chaplain assistant director at South Mercy Hospital, and Reverend that is working a full time at Roswell Park. Conclusions were drawn regarding the expectations different site directors.

The Spiritual Care Assessment was implemented at Roswell Park for a period of one year. The chaplains charted all the patient intervention electronically every day. The effectiveness of the spiritual care assessment for palliative care patients was evaluated for one year. Palliative care patients were visited almost every day. "Clear, precise and generous communications is essential to a good-patient-doctor relationship. Especially with serious of life –threatening illness, your doctor must be ready to "go extra mile "in time of crisis, to ensure that you have been told and have heard and understood the diagnosis, the treatment options with all the implications and the prognosis for your recovery. (Seguin, 1992)

This project was completed in December 2019.

Chapter Reflections

- How do you feel about the evaluation of Spiritual Care by the chaplains?
- Explain the personal spiritual care in you as a chaplain?
- What is the reason for the evaluation in both areas, such as: spiritual and palliative care?
- Who has proven to be the Master of Assessments, as read?
- Do you think it is necessary for the chaplain to make a personal evaluation of his spiritual level every day?

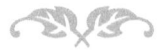

CHAPTER 5

NARRATIVE OF INITIATIVE IMPLEMENTATION

This initiative is the road map to success. Roswell Park is the exact place for this to happen with committed chaplains and great support from the administration. Every morning, after reviewing the case load for the day, chaplains arrived at the rooms to start the most important task at the beginning of the interview. Using the Assessment Interview tool, they accurately grasped the most relevant needs of the patients. The tool helped them discover important information about religious choice, factors of lifestyle and action, trauma, and medical treatment, for example. One of my patients was a 33-year-old Caucasian woman. She was a Caucasian single mother. During The first overview assessment, I saw a person with serious physical problems and a general belief in God or a Higher Power. She was not interested in talking but seemed very secure. Her room was dark, and she seemed to be in poor health. During the second assessment, the patient mentioned the word "anxious." That marked the beginning of a Pandora's Box of her concerns. The patient opened her heart and started describing her entire life from the time she was seven years old. Her father had abused her sexually for many years. When she grew up, she was involved in heavy drinking and the use of tobacco and heroin. She had a 12-year-old daughter and was a single mother. Because of her addictions, the patient had attempted to kill herself many times. The last time, she considered stepping down into the Niagara River. The patient mentioned that she was seeing a psychiatrist and a counselor and was controlling her depression and anxiety disorder through medication. She has already been tobacco- and drug-free for six months.

After I assessed the patient, she was able to present a more practical, accurate, and healthier follow-up. Assessment is important for both chaplain and the patient. There is the case of another patient who seemed to be a very strong man, a civil engineer from Texas. During the assessment, in reference to family, he mentioned that he had just come from Texas one month before. He had no family, no clergy support, and no coworker support. This patient was facing a possible major surgery a few hours later. After a pleasant conversation, he indicated that his belief system was Christian. However, he felt a great sense of grief. He missed his family and friends, but the chaplain's visits seemed to give him a sense of communion, relationship, and care.

When the project was implemented every chaplain and chaplain aids were ready to take action. Chaplain researcher provided them with total 34 questions, to be answered according to their possibility, understanding and experience. The advantage of the group is the constant relationship with palliative care patients. Everyone was trained to develop the survey in the time and the way they believed was the most personally convenient the survey itself provided the pathway to follow. The first question has a close relationship with the following question and the last question can be enough also matched with the first question. For example complying about Environment survey with 9 questions. Chaplain have the time to test their ability to interact with different genders. Some of them responded that they just preferred to visit female patients other on the other side male patients. Oher have difficult to visit LGTB community patients. And preferred to delegate that responsibility to others who feels more comfortable. Also the kind of religion for some chaplains could be an encounter of a problematic environment, some of them prefer just to visit their own line of religion, although for most of the chaplains special the one who are a fulltime, it seems unreal. This test provide to chaplain to create means or exercise their skills how to share spiritual care with patient that have received the news of negative diagnosis. The struggle between patient and family are real and painful. Or the ones whose chances to survive are minimum. Columns of support with total 10 questions, embrace questions that makes chaplains reflect in their own strengths regarding how they are feeling when pastoring patients from other denominations that their own. Also allows to analyze their relationship with the medical team (Nurses, Physicians, Nurses aide and the administration. For example in the Soarian Program are contemplated 14 religions options: Catholics, Protestants, Christians, Hindu, Jehovah Witnesses, Jewish, Latter Day Saints, Muslim, Native American Indian, Unitarian Universalist, Buddhist, etc., others like Meditech, and Crescendo have different way to record religious worldview. Every chaplain has the opportunity to show their skills during patient intervention. Also let chaplains in this part of the survey weight how the medical team views the Spiritual Support as a vital part of the patient recovery. How important is the presence of the chaplain in the patient's room. Support from the Spiritual team, program director is also evaluated and the most important, this part of the survey allows the chaplain to see his grow during the ministering at the site. One more and important point in this part of the survey is the relationship of the Chaplain with the patient's family, patient's friend, and sometimes with the clergy that has close ties with the patient. Scholarity (9 questions), was implemented to discover the level of education of the caregiver, dedication to continue education, resources that are available for the chaplain and also to provide patients request. But also the dynamic inside the pastoral team that can be positive or negative. And Preparedness (7 questions) goes direct over the chaplain's intellectual and experience preparation and readiness to perform his ministry, is well known experienced chaplains will deliver broad branches of care than the novelties. This are also analyze the places where chaplain were acting in the past, and how they can resolve unexpected issues that is common to see during Spiritual Care visitation... In the group many of the chaplains are professionals (6) and rather ones who are nonprofessionals (24) but they are people of a deep ministerial experience either in church or as a layman leading huge spiritual service projects inside their communities. All the surveys were mailed or sometimes were personally provided personally. The survey was prepared exclusively for the Spiritual Care Team members. No patients were involved in the survey. Chaplains, were selected because of the daily contact with patients, patient's family and other medical team. Data collection was received by mail or directly in person. Closed envelope. At the end of the survey when all the information was collected we applied the Likert-Type Scales (Graphic Scales) to select the responses and grouping them and obtaining the numbers that will allow to develop the percentages and ratios that will put in evidence the importance of the responses in determinate areas of research. "A Likert Scale is a used to measure the attitude wherein the respondents are asked to indicate the level of agreement or disagreement with the statements related to the stimulus objects"(busssinessjargon, 2020).

Chapter Reflections

- How important is planning for chaplains' activities in the morning?
- Why is constant relationship with palliative care patients necessary?
- How important is the chaplain's relationship with the patient's family and friends in the survey?
- Do you think that in order to carry out a project, the attitude of support between chaplains and their assistants is very good?
- What is the patient's reaction after an evaluation?
- Could you explain a personal experience when evaluating a patient?

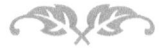

CHAPTER 6
EVALUATION AND LEARNINGS

Method of Evaluation

Personal surveys (Appendix A) were distributed to all the chaplains who were in contact with palliative care patients after having received approval from both the Roswell Park Comprehensive Cancer Center IRB and the Andrews University IRB. The survey was composed of Environment, Sources of Support, Academic Training, and Preparation. We tried to think in a broader context "to ensure that research participation [was] accessible to all" and so that flexible "recruitment methods that permit adaptation to specific needs arising out of health status, level of involvement with services, culture, and socioeconomic status" (Rugkasa & Canvin, 2011, p. 132) were employed.

The chaplains were provided with the surveys (34 total). All of them had contact with palliative care patients in a daily basis. When they come in the morning shift or afternoon shift or weekend shift they will found on the spiritual care department desk their assignations that include number of the floor, patients selected by time to enter in the system (New Admits) or patients that stay more time in the hospital (Follow-Ups). The one who already are admitted into de Palliative Care Program they will appear in the Patient

Census Report highlighted by pink color. The one who ae new admits and follow -ups they will cheeked using blue or blank pencil. And then go the assigned floor used palliative care assessment to get information after. Having all the chaplains (N=30) received a copy of the informed consent which was evidence based to avoid any thing that could harm them or the patients. 27 have returned with the survey done. The attrition number was 3. Research has found that

> Freely given informed consent to participation is the ethical cornerstone of research in health care. However, in mental health settings, there are many patients who lack the capacity to give such consent to participate in research. There is an abundance of guidance now available on how researchers might think about this issue and the Royal College of Psychiatrists has also recently reviewed its guidance to members about the ethics of research. (Adshead, 2012, p. 141)

I explained them about the use and purpose of the survey, to discover the areas in Palliative Care Assessment that will need to be improved. And it took more than a month for the surveys to be returned. All the surveys were anonymous, they just need to read and execute the survey and the results were entered exactly as they were given.

Results and Analysis of Evaluation

Table 1 shows the male and female patients by percentage that each chaplain was responsible for.

Table 1
Case Load

Chaplain	% Male Patients	% Female Patients
1	50	50
2	50	50
3	50	50
4	50	50
5	40	60
6	40	60

The Environment part of the survey (Table 2) had nine questions that produced the following results that demonstrated my personal assessment of the chaplain-patient interactions during visitation: In question 4 concerning receptivity, 67% of the respondents agreed that Boomer patients were more open to chaplain visits than Millennials. In question 6 concerning religious receptivity, 50% said there was no difference; one chaplain responded, "Just Catholics"; and another chaplain said that Protestant patients were more receptive than Catholics. On question 7 that was specific about certain religious groups being more open than others, 2 of the surveyed chaplains mentioned that they found it difficult to minister to Jewish and Muslim patients. The rest of the chaplains found no difference. Question 9 that had to do with handling discouraged patients, 100% of those surveyed responded that they had a positive way to handle the specific situation.

Table 2
Environment

Negative Outcome	Listening	Comfort	Encourage	Listening	Faith	Empathy
PPre-s/Pos	NN/A	NN/A	PPos	PPos	NN/A	NN/A
Difficult	N/A	N/A	Same	Jewish	Non	Muslim
Receptive P NonP	Catholics	Same	Same	Protestant	N/A	Same
Marital Status	Most Married	N/A	Married	Both	N/A	Either
MB	Same	Same	Boomers	Boomers	Boomers	Boomers
Ages	50+	0-Grave	Seniors	25-85	45-65	45+
Comfort MF	Same	Same	Both	Same	Same	Either
Case Load						
MF	50% 50%	50% 50%	50% 50%	50% 50%	40% 60%	40% 60%

There were nine questions to be answered in the Sources of Support part of the survey (Table 3). In answering question 3, 43% of the surveyed chaplains said that the medical team fully understood their function, but only 57% somewhat understood. This indicates that most of the medical team still needed to be trained in this area (question 3). For question 4, the chaplains said that 86.6% of the medical team respected their presence in the patient's room, allowing the spiritual visit to be more fruitful. One chaplain said the opposite. When they responded to question 6, all the chaplains surveyed said that they had positive and efficient support from the staff chaplains. The last noticeable response in the area of Sources of Support concerned the Spiritual Care Department. Forty-three percent did not respond to the question, while the 57% who did respond suggested that the department needs to have more retreats, mental health days, more proficient scheduling, and more presence in the clinic settings.

The next part of the survey analyzed was Academic Training (Table 4). This part also had nine questions to demonstrate the level of academic training the chaplains doing spiritual assessment at the hospital had. At this point, question 1 of the survey shows that, on average, the academic training of the staff chaplain was seven years. Question 6 showed that 30% of the chaplains have a Master's in Divinity, while 42% have a degree in Pastoral Ministry, and 28% have other degrees. One Chaplain has a PhD. The chaplains spend an average of 2-22 minutes in the patients' rooms (Question 7).

The fourth area of the survey, Preparation (Table 5), had seven questions. The average experience of the staff chaplains was 11 years (question 1). Concerning this experience, 57% had experience in settings such as hospitals, prisons, hospices, and so on (question 2). Question 4 asked whether their work required knowledge of human psychology, and 71% said that doing chaplaincy in general requires that knowledge. Responses to question 6 show that 57% had CPE preparation, but one lay chaplain only requested more information about CPE. Question 7 had to do with how the chaplains react to unwelcoming patients. The responses show that 86% of the chaplains treated them with dignity and one did not respond to the question. In regard to these results, various studies done by other researchers confirm that a chaplain's preparation and time are also factors that can affect the attention to patients facing cancer. "Barriers to spiritual

Table 3
Sources of Support

Personal Grow	Yes	In many ways	Yes	Yes	Yes	N/A
Patient Request	Yes	Yes	Yes	Yes	Yes	Yes
Family Interaction	receptive	Open	included	respectful	Joyful	Very well
Staff Support	Must supporting	We all get along	Positive	Positively	Efficiently	Positive
PC Improvement	Session thoughts	N/A	N/A	Retreats, mental health days	Scheduling	N/A
Med Team Respect	Yes	No	Mostly	Yes	Yes	Very much
Med Team Understands	Yes	Most of them	Yes	Somewhat	I try to	
stay out of						
their way	yes					
Interaction with Non	Respect	N/A	N/A	Non-		
judgmental	Pray to God					
and not						
to Jesus	N/A					
Christian %	100%	All faiths	Mostly	No	90%	100%

Table 4
Academic Training

Funeral Activity?	yes	yes	yes	yes	no	yes
Process of Dying?	yes	yes	yes	yes	yes	yes
How Long	30 min	As needed	2-25 min	20-30 min	2-15 min	As needed
Higher Education	Pastoral Ministry	Pastoral Ministry	Building trades	MDiv	History	MDiv/PhD
Pursuing a Degree	Yes	No	No	N/A	No	No
Provided Sources	Yes	Yes	Yes	No	Yes	Yes
Yearly Training	yes	yes	yes	yes	no	yes
Years of Preparation	20	26	10	4	24	16
Professional	yes	no	yes	no	yes	yes
Unwelcome Patients	Respect	Respect	Gentle	Thanks	N/A	Support

Table 5
Preparation

CPE Units	Zero	4	Zero	4	Zero	1
Psychological/ Spiritual Approach	Spiritual	Both	Both	Behavioral	Spiritual	N/A
Needed to Know Human Psychology	Yes	Yes	Yes	Yes	Experience	Counseling
Comfort in Assignments	Yes	Yes	Yes	Yes	N/A	yes
Other Settings Exp	No	Yes	No	Yes	No	Yes
Years as Chaplain	1.5	26	9	4	Many	13

care include lack of time, personal, cultural or institutional factors, and professional educational needs" (Edwards, Pang, Shiu, & Chan, 2010, p. 753).

In reference to the activity of the staff chaplains on a daily basis, we did a tracking to know exactly what was happening during visits to the palliative population of Roswell Hospital while still stressing the activity directed toward palliative care patients for 19 days during October 2018. The following were the results:

As noted above, a record I made every day at Roswell Park of those with in-patient status. One month's observation demonstrated that there are more women in-patients than men. The floor that had the most patients was floor 6, with an average of 5 palliative care patients per day. The ICU had one per day. This study also demonstrated that females facing cancer were younger (average age of 54) than males (average age of 60).

Regarding spiritual care intervention by Religion, this research (October 2018-January 2019) found that chaplains visited 42% Catholic patients, (a total of 621). Non-denominational patients (249) were the second largest number of patients with 17% of total number of patients visited for that period. Numbers of those self-identifying according to various other Christian affiliations are as follows: Christians (133), 9%; Protestants (112), 7%; Methodists, 6%; Baptists, 5%; Episcopalians/Lutherans, 3%; and others, 1%. Jews, Jehovah's Witnesses, Muslims, and Buddhists are 0.6% of the population.

My Transformation as a Ministry Professional

I received my first call to work as a pastor in the northern area of Peru in 1982. The call to the ministry was rooted in my life and the life of my family from that time. I never doubted my call, even in moments of struggle or when the Conference Board reassigned me to a new field, and I had to leave an area I loved and had been successfully doing ministry for many years. I remember that my first field of work after graduation from seminary was in the big city of Chiclayo, located in the northeast area of Peru on the shores of the Pacific Ocean. This place was a real blessing for me especially because my mentor was one of the most experienced ministers working in that area. I learned the first steps of doing ministerial business from him, and those lessons have lasted throughout my life. My mentor started as a church pastor, then became district pastor, and finally president of the conference. This gave me the assurance that God was leading my life and was preparing me to new and more challenging actions in the future. His guiding experience led me to understand the wide horizon of the pastoral ministry as spiritual leader and counselor. I grew as a minister, nurtured by my mentor's daily family devotions and prayers, weekly planning meetings, as well as the great support of the churches that had been assigned to me.

After one year in the city of Chiclayo, the Conference Board considered me to be a primary candidate to reopen a new field in a remote area of the country called Rodriguez de Mendoza. When I received the letter signed by the President of the Conference with my new assignment, I felt stunned. The first thing I did was to pray with my wife so we could find the city of Rodriguez de Mendoza on the map of Peru. My search was unsuccessful because the city was even not named in the most popular maps of Peru in 1983. In consultation with Conference executives, the Secretary of the Conference gave me a list of possible church members. Those members were in a long-neglected (20 years) field, but the Conference leadership was secure in the belief that my youthful impulse and fresh ministering strategies would make the new district headquarters a reality in that remote area. I still remember how difficult that change was for my family and me. I found the Adventist congregation in the Mendoza area had been scattered many years before by a group of Reformists (supported by dissidents of the Adventist movement in the United States), and there were no more official Adventists members anymore. Going from a big city with churches full of very active members, very appealing buildings, and vibrant enthusiasm in every program of the church to facing a big challenge where there was no church and those remaining were just nominal members was an unusual experience for me. Most of the members I found identified themselves as members of the Seventh-day Adventist Reform Movement. The place for a possible central church building was in the middle of the private property without any street designation. I had to open it and name it. However, every challenge I found in that place was a very rewarding experience in developing my personal ministry. Things like opening streets, weekly construction fairs, South American fund support, and aggressive family Bible studies and outreach evangelism campaigns were the clues to expanding the gospel in my new area. Rodriguez de Mendoza was the place that provided me invaluable ministry training, but also the place where God blessed me with one of my beloved daughters. Rodriguez de Mendoza was the place where I really found the reason for the mission in my life. This place was not unlike Patmos (far away from civilization) where John was sent and was the opportunity for me to grow in every area of my life and to nurture my family. Villages where no Adventist church where found was where I had to build a new church. If there was no Adventist congregation, I had to create one. If it was necessary to create access to a place of worship and a health-related center (my wife was a registered nurse), then I had to do it. It was the opportunity to be really creative, an expert in public relations, counselor, church planter, front-line evangelist, trainer, town council member, traveler, and more. Years later, when I had to move to other geographic areas, I used this experience to resolve church-related issues with better skills and preparation.

Working in areas of Peru from the north to the south was a rewarding experience that prepared me for the big move, coming to the United States. I came as a literature evangelist to the Northeastern Conference of New York. I had done this kind of work as a theology student for many years, but now I had to do it as my principal ministry in New England. Being constantly in contact with new families as prospective customers of our denominational books prepared me to assimilate the American culture (and the language, too). It was full of challenges, and at the same time, was a completely different arena from the South American viewpoint and lifestyle. One of the challenges was to learn a new way of religious life. In the area where I started my ministry in New Bedford, Massachusetts, I found that every congregation had rented a beautiful building from another religious denomination, but there was not much attendance at church services. My first interaction with an Adventist church was to find a perfect building church that would hold 200 people, but I counted just 20 members (including children) during the worship service. This was the reality of the church back in the 90s when I started my new journey in America. Faith and perseverance were the ingredients to put to those congregations of Dominican Republic, Puerto Rican, and Brazilian immigrants. Another very important cultural shock was to discover that I was a member of the Hispanic community. I never knew this particular designation until a member of the church advised me that there were other Seventh-day Adventist congregations in the area. A Portuguese Church, an African-American Church, an American Church, and so on. I had to learn very quickly of the changes that give the Seventh-day Adventist Church an opportunity to integrate into a church full of varieties in cultures, ways to worship, and visions. God led me to be part of the potential to help grow these congregations exploding in hope, mission work, and desire to see their congregations expanded to the greatest degree possible.

After years of working as a literature evangelist, the New York Conference invited me to be a church planter in Buffalo, New York, where I still live today. I worked in Buffalo for many years as a church planter and God provided me with the necessary tools to establish a new congregation in the southern area of the city that shines as a lighthouse to the people who need to learn the truth and wait for the Second Coming of the Lord. Eight years ago my ministry, I had the opportunity to become a chaplain. When I received approval to take the CPE course in a center managed by the Catholic Sisters of Charity that run many schools and hospitals in the area of Western New York, I never thought this new area would change my approach. When the time to start the chaplaincy internship became a reality, I was very afraid because I did not know that a hospital setting could be an amazing place to provide spiritual nurture and hope to people. However, I soon understood that "prayer" chaplains are valuable in helping to meet the pastoral care needs of the spiritual family.

> Serving as a Prayer Chaplain is a volunteer opportunity for those members who are truly looking to take the next step in the development of their spiritual maturity, and who are willing to make a high level of commitment in their spiritual growth. (Asato, 2019, para. 6).

I then understood that God had a deeper purpose for me— being part of the chaplaincy team. There were people, many of them not members of my congregation, who were thirsting for spiritual help. After training of four units of CPE, I started enjoying a new ministry in Roman Catholic hospitals. At the same time, the horizon of my ministry was broadened. There was no doubt that God's call was in that area of service. I soon discovered that chaplains try to find any means to supply the spiritual needs of the patient without any barriers. As a minister involved in the growth of my church, I never realized that people outside my congregation, like hospital patients, were also waiting for me and also deserve to hear the message of hope.

Chaplaincy gave me that new opportunity to serve my community faith, relate to my conference colleagues, and at the same time, interact with other community faith leaders and serve the "other sheep of the flock." Sometimes I ask myself what the difference is between my calling as a minister, pastoring my congregation, and ministering as a hospital chaplain. The answer was not easy to find, but one day, I found this statement that portrayed what was on my mind: both callings are wonderful in a person's life and both are desperately needed, but they are very different in ministry, and chaplaincy needed still more preparation. A pastor's ministry deals mainly with in-reach or, shall we say, is church-based, whereas a chaplain's ministry deals mainly with outreach and is community-based. A simple definition of a chaplain is a minister in the workplace. In other words, chaplains have a home church they attend, but their church is actually outside the walls of the church building. Chaplains serve people of all faiths. Going to the Bible, for example, I found that after listening to Nehemiah, the king asked him,

> "What do you request from me?" Again, Nehemiah prayed, and then he said, "If it pleases the king may I have letters to the governors of all the regions so they allow me to safely pass through until I come to Judah . . . also may I have a letter to Asaph, keeper of the king's forest, so that he must give me all the timber to rebuild the gates." (Neh 2:7, 8)

The king granted Nehemiah's request and ultimately, the walls and gates were rebuilt, and the people were secure. The point of this story is that God used a pagan king, Artaxerxes, to see that His work (the rebuilding of the wall around Jerusalem) was accomplished by God's people. God used pagan resources for kingdom purposes. As we understand from this passage of Scripture, Nehemiah was the bridge God used to see that the work was done. He not only did God's work, but also did it with the king's blessing and support. That is the protection a chaplain has. Part of the chaplain's ministry is to be a bridge between the secular and the sacred. My job as a chaplain inside a non-Adventist setting is like the work of Nehemiah—a small light that brightens a corner of the world that would otherwise not be cared for and would be in darkness. Now they have additional insight to help them grasp possibilities that will carry them to the kingdom of heaven.

Chapter Reflection

- Do you agree with personal surveys (as a mode of research) conducted by chaplains on palliative care patients?
- What is the cornerstone in research ethics, in health care?
- Do you think that when one surrenders himself to God, he places his children in the place where they can gain experience for future work?
- Explain your personal, intellectual, practical experience in chaplaincy work.
- How much did this book help you to learn about the work of a chaplain dedicated to palliative care patients?

Verbatim

Do an exercise of this tool to explain your experience during the interaction with a patient, use the model that is most familiar to you.

CHAPTER 7
EMMY-NOMINATED LIFE RECORDED

A Palliative Care Approach to Preserving a Patient's Life Story

In the realm of healthcare where science, spirituality, compassion and artistic creativity converge, a revolutionary program called "Life Recorded" has emerged, transforming the landscape of the Palliative and Spiritual Care Departments at Roswell Park Comprehensive Cancer Center. More than a compilation of medical records and treatment plans, Life Recorded encapsulates the essence of individuals facing the challenging journey of cancer by recording their stories of cancer, family, and life. This chapter explores the inception, implementation, and profound impact of Life Recorded in the cancer hospital setting, emphasizing its multimodal methods that have made a huge impact on the lives of patients, their families, their care teams, and the greater cancer community. Coauthor of this book, Paul Spitale, PhD, has run the Life Recorded Program for nearly four years.

Life Recorded is a program originally intended to record the stories of patients, their families, their caregivers, doctors, nurses, anyone associated with Roswell Park, and anyone else touched by cancer.

With the use of audio, video, and other methods, Life Recorded has archived over 400 pieces since its inception. The integration of technology plays a pivotal role in ensuring the accessibility of Life Recorded to patients beyond the physical confines of the cancer center. Remote recording sessions, virtual support groups, and online resources extend the program's reach, particularly for patients who may face physical and/or geographical challenges. This technological integration aligns with the broader trend of telehealth in healthcare delivery. One of the strengths of Life Recorded lies in its ability to tailor approaches to individual needs. Recognizing that each patient's journey is unique, the program ensures a personalized and flexible recording process. This adaptability is crucial in accommodating diverse cultural backgrounds, belief systems, and preferences, fostering a sense of inclusivity and respect. Through Life Recorded, patients are empowered to shape their own legacies. The program provides a structured and supportive environment for individuals to express their identity, values, and stories, allowing them to be active participants in their lives, the lives of their family, and how they will be remembered.

Life Recorded's multimodal methods contribute to holistic support for patients in palliative care. By addressing not only the physical but also the emotional, spiritual, and existential aspects of their lives, the program becomes a cornerstone in enhancing the overall quality of life during the final stages of the cancer journey. Life Recorded serves as a powerful advocate for comprehensive palliative care. Its success underscores the importance of integrating psychosocial and existential aspects into the broader spectrum of healthcare. Life Recorded does not focus solely on the illness experience but encourages patients to share narratives beyond their diagnosis. By capturing the richness of individuals' lives, the program transcends the confines of illness, celebrating achievements, passions, and moments of joy. This broader approach reinforces the idea that a person is not defined solely by their medical condition but by the entirety of their existence.

History and Inception of Life Recorded

The genesis of Life Recorded can be traced back to 2014, where compassionate visionaries within the Spiritual Care Department at Roswell Park saw beyond the conventional boundaries of patient care. Driven by the understanding that healing extends beyond physical ailments, the Director of Spiritual Care engaged the assistance of a national storytelling program to formulate a customized platform at Roswell Park. Within the context of Roswell Park, the Spiritual Care Department plays a pivotal role in ensuring the success of Life Recorded. The department serves as the nurturing ground for the program, providing the necessary spiritual and emotional support for patients and their families. Chaplains, counselors, and other spiritual care providers collaborate to integrate the program seamlessly into the holistic care provided at the cancer center. In 2014, members from the international storytelling show "StoryCorps" ascended on Roswell Park Comprehensive Cancer Center to begin what would be a decade-long journey to successfully archive patient narratives. Little did anyone know at the time the tremendous impact the program would have on the lives of patients, families, caregivers, hospital staff, and the public. Until 2019 the program delivered just what it promised: to give patients a voice to record their thoughts, dreams, and messages for loved ones.

It was not until 2020 that the program would take an incredibly creative, inspiring, and impactful direction. That is when Paul Spitale, Ph.D., a visionary researcher, educator, and filmmaker with a passion for holistic patient care, spearheaded the evolution of Life Recorded. Witnessing the profound impact of shared narratives on patient well-being, he envisioned a program that would offer more than just a patient's medical journey and documentation. He believed in the power of storytelling to heal, connect, and inspire. The idea germinated during a conversation with a patient, Andrew Posner (a pseudonym), whose eyes sparked with the depth of unspoken stories. Andrew's wish to be remembered beyond his illness planted the seed for a program that would celebrate lives, not just document diseases. Dr. Spitale gathered a diverse team of professionals – videographers, writers, artists, and therapists – to create vivacity in what was seen as the resurgence of Life Recorded at Roswell Park Comprehensive Cancer Center.

The idea was not merely to document the medical aspects of a patient's journey but to capture the story, the history, the soul, and the essence of life that each individual brings to the world. From 2014 to 2020, the program staff and volunteers recorded and average of 20-30 audio and video interviews per year. It was not until 2020, when the Covid pandemic struck the program dead in the water, that Paul Spitale, Ph.D. was hired to revive the program. Since Dr. Spitale's takeover, Life Recorded has been internationally recognized, garnered several awards and grants, and even received an Emmy nomination for its documentary "When I See You: A Cancer Patient's Journey" which can be viewed on YouTube (youtube.com/watch?v=OtDXVPUN6wE). More importantly however, it has archived over 300 multimodal pieces in under three years in the form of audio and video interviews, musical recordings, poetry, short stories, paintings, sketches, as well as award-winning documentary films. Dr. Spitale has recruited a multidisciplinary team comprised of chaplains, physicians, nurses, psychologists, social workers, researchers, and artists who together have advanced the program to redefine supportive and palliative care.

Implementation of Multimodal Methods

Audio Narratives

At the heart of Life Recorded are audio narratives, where patients are encouraged to share their life stories, memories, and reflections. Trained professionals conduct interviews, guiding patients through a journey of self-expression. The soothing cadence of a patient's voice narrating their life story creates an intimate connection, fostering a sense of comfort and closure. Audio narratives take the form of unscripted interviews and conversations as well as scripted accounts that chronicle patients' lives. Other audio narratives have been implemented as well. For example, one 79-year-old patient had written his memoirs at the request of his family. He was not completely satisfied with the final product, so Dr. Spitale suggested they create an audiobook from them. After pulling from his vast resources, the patient was gifted with a professionally-prepared audiobook, narrated by an award-winning voiceover actor, worthy of streaming quality. These audio narratives serve not only as personal healing channels for patients but also as tangible gifts for their families.

Video Chronicles

Visual storytelling plays a pivotal role in the Life Recorded program. With the help of video recordings, patients can convey their emotions, experiences, and aspirations in a powerful and tangible way. The camera becomes a conduit for unspoken words, capturing the nuances of their expressions, smiles, and tears. Body language and facial expression dictates the visual modality. Dr. Spitale has also enlisted the help of Roswell Park's creative team in filming, directing, and editing award-winning documentary films that chronicle moments in patients' lives. For example, a 21-year-old patient with late-stage IV metastasized cancer was interested in leaving a message for his three-year-old daughter. Dr. Spitale interviewed him via video and found that the patient was a musician and songwriter. Dr. Spitale suggested he write a song for his daughter for her to have for the rest of her life. The patient agreed and with the help of a local recording studio, the patient was able to record her a beautiful song. The recording session was filmed and the process was produced into an award-winning behind-the-scenes documentary. These videos serve not only as a therapeutic outlet for patients but also as invaluable legacies for their loved ones.

Artistic Expression

Recognizing the therapeutic power of art, Life Recorded incorporates various forms of artistic expression. With aid from the Roswell Park "Art Heals" Gallery and the Resource Center, patients are provided with art supplies and encouraged to create visual representations of their experiences, feelings and memories. One patient, a 35-year-old male artist had massed a volume of artistic works dating back to the 3rd grade. Life Recorded staff collected some of his works and presented them at a gallery-like art show posthumously. Family, friends, caregivers, and hospital staff showed up in droves for a standing-room-only event to view and honor the patients' works. Whether painting, drawing, or sculpting, this creative outlet becomes a source of solace and self-discovery for patients facing the challenges of cancer.

Written Reflections

In the written dimension of Life Recorded, patients are given the opportunity to pen down their thoughts, reflections, and even letters to their loved ones. The written word becomes a timeless medium through which patients can convey their deepest emotions, fears, and gratitude. As a certified writing professor, Dr. Spitale holds a semi-quarterly journaling workshop using his published workbook "Journaling for Purpose" to allow people to learn how to express themselves and use journaling proactively. These written reflections are not only therapeutic for the patients but also serve as profound mementos for their families. Additionally, many patients express themselves in other forms of writing they find more comfortable. Some patients are published authors themselves. Life Recorded provides them with an outlet to express themselves in writing.

Narratives Beyond Illness

Life Recorded does not focus solely on the illness experience but encourages patients to share narratives beyond their diagnosis. By capturing the richness of individuals' lives, the program transcends the confines of illness, celebrating achievements, passions, creativity, and moments of joy. This broader approach reinforces the idea that a person is not defined solely by their medical condition but by the entirety of their existence. Life Recorded places a strong emphasis on celebrating the diversity of human experiences. The program acknowledges that each person's journey is unique, shaped by cultural backgrounds, beliefs, and personal histories. Cultural competence is woven into the fabric of Life Recorded, ensuring that the program is inclusive and respectful of diverse perspectives on life, death, and legacy.

Challenges

Implementing a program like Life Recorded is not without its challenges. The sensitive nature of recording personal stories requires vigilant ethical considerations and privacy safeguards. Initial resistance may arise from both healthcare providers and patients due to concerns about emotional distress, time constraints, or the intrusion of privacy. Overcoming these challenges requires a gradual introduction of the program, comprehensive training, and ongoing support for healthcare professionals. Life Recorded implements strict protocols to ensure that the dignity and confidentiality of patients are preserved. Informed consent processes are thorough, and patients are given the agency to dictate the boundaries of their narratives. Additionally, cybersecurity measures are employed to protect the recorded materials, recognizing the profound responsibility of safeguarding the legacies entrusted to the program. Striking a balance between the desire to capture authentic narratives and respecting the sensitivity of the situation is an ongoing process that requires continuous evaluation and adaptation. Addressing these concerns ensures that Life Recorded becomes a welcomed and integral component of palliative care.

Fostering Dignity, Empowerment, Legacy and Memory

Life Recorded transcends the traditional narrative of illness, offering patients a platform to reclaim their narratives. In the face of terminal diagnoses, patients often experience a loss of control over their lives. Life Recorded empowers them to assert their agency, fostering a sense of dignity and autonomy throughout their journey. Palliative care is not just about the end of life; it is about preserving the richness of a person's existence. Life Recorded plays a pivotal role in a cancer hospital by addressing the holistic needs of patients facing the challenges of a life-threatening illness. Its importance lies in enhancing the quality of life for individuals affected by cancer, focusing on relieving pain, managing symptoms, and providing emotional and spiritual support. Unlike curative treatments, palliative care is not limited by the stage of the disease and can be integrated alongside ongoing therapies. This specialized care that Life Recorded provides helps alleviate mental and emotional stress by providing an outlet for patients to express themselves.

Many patients have described their sessions as "therapeutic" and "healing." Recording sessions often attend to the psychological and social dimensions of the patient's experience, fostering a sense of dignity and control. Life Recorded extends its embrace to include the family members and caregivers of patients By embracing a patient-centered approach, Life Recorded ensures that individuals and their families are actively involved in storytelling, fostering open communication and creating a supportive environment during a challenging journey. Recognizing the interconnectedness of lives, the program encourages the recording of shared stories, capturing the collective experiences of those who stand alongside the patient. This holistic approach not only provides support for the family but also fosters a sense of unity and understanding. Ultimately, the integration of Life Recorded in palliative care emphasizes compassionate and comprehensive care that goes beyond medical treatments, promoting a dignified and comfortable experience for patients grappling with the complexities of cancer. Life Recorded ensures that the legacy of each patient is not confined to medical charts and treatment plans. Instead, it becomes a living testament to their unique journey, allowing family members to cherish and celebrate the life that was lived.

Life Recorded serves as a catalyst for cultivating empathy within the healthcare profession. By immersing healthcare providers in the multifaceted narratives of patients and their families, the program fosters a deeper understanding of the emotional and psychological dimensions of illness. This empathic connection, in turn, enhances the quality of care provided, creating a more compassionate and supportive healthcare environment.

Patient-Centered Care

Life Recorded amplifies the principles of patient-centered care by placing the patient's narrative at the forefront. Through the program, healthcare providers gain a more comprehensive understanding of the individual behind the illness, enabling them to tailor care plans that resonate with the patient's values and preferences. Engaging in the multimodal methods offered by Life Recorded has a profound impact on the emotional well-being of patients. It provides a cathartic release, allowing individuals to express and process their emotions in a supportive environment. This emotional outlet contributes significantly to a patient's overall quality of life during palliative care.

Extending the Embrace: Recording Family Members and Caregivers

Caregivers often find themselves on an emotionally taxing journey alongside their loved ones. Life Recorded acknowledges the pivotal role played by caregivers and extends its support by recording their experiences, fears, and triumphs. By recognizing the caregiver's narrative, the program fosters a supportive environment for those who are providing invaluable support to patients. The journey through cancer is not an isolated experience but a collective one. As such, the program extends its embrace to include the narratives of patients' family members and caregivers. This extension recognizes the interconnectedness of lives and provides a platform for all those involved to share their stories, fears, and triumphs.

Continuous Improvement and Feedback

The success of Life Recorded relies on an iterative process of improvement based on patient feedback and healthcare provider experiences. Regular feedback methods are utilized to understand the emotional impact on patients, ensuring that the program remains a source of comfort rather than distress. Continuous improvement also involves training healthcare providers to navigate the sensitive nature of recording sessions and ensuring that ethical considerations are prioritized.

Building Bridges with the Community

Recognizing the importance of community engagement, Life Recorded extends its reach beyond the hospital setting. The program actively seeks collaborations with local artists, community organizations, and volunteers to expand its reach. Art exhibits showcasing patients' creations, community workshops, and awareness campaigns have become integral components of Life Recorded. By building bridges with the community, the program aims to destigmatize discussions around palliative care and encourage a more open dialogue about legacy-building and end-of-life experiences. Community outreach initiatives, such as workshops and public exhibitions, aim to destigmatize discussions surrounding death and dying, contributing to a more compassionate and informed society.

Life Recorded serves as a practical model for cultivating empathy and patient-centered care in the next generation of healthcare providers. To maximize the impact of Life Recorded, international collaborations and knowledge exchange initiatives are essential. By sharing experiences, best practices, and cultural insights, the program can adapt to different healthcare systems and societal norms. These collaborations also foster a sense of global solidarity in recognizing the universal need for compassionate end-of-life care.

Global Impact and Future Collaborations

As the success stories of Life Recorded echo through the healthcare community, there is a growing interest in adopting similar programs worldwide. International collaborations are underway to share best practices, develop standardized ethical guidelines, and adapt the program to diverse cultural contexts. The vision is to create a global network where the essence of each individual's life is honored and preserved, regardless of geographic or cultural differences. Life Recorded Program Coordinator Dr. Paul Spitale is consistently meeting with international organizers and constantly looking to create meaningful global partnerships.

The Role of Technology

In an era dominated by technological advancements, Life Recorded leverages cutting-edge tools to enhance its impact. Currently, the program director is looking to experiment with virtual reality (VR) experiences, for instance, to enable patients to immerse themselves in meaningful virtual environments, creating additional avenues for expression. Moreover, technology facilitates the remote participation of family members and allows for the seamless integration of Life Recorded into telemedicine practices, ensuring accessibility for patients in various settings.

Research and Evaluation: Measuring Impact and Improving Care

An essential component of Life Recorded's journey at Roswell Park is a commitment to ongoing research and evaluation. The program collects and analyzes data to measure its impact on patients' well-being, family dynamics, and the overall quality of the program within palliative care. Insights gained from these studies contribute to continuous improvement, ensuring that the program remains responsive to the evolving needs of patients and their families. Continuous research and data collection contribute to a growing body of evidence supporting the positive impact of Life Recorded on patients, families, and caregivers.

Reflections and Future Prospects

The journey of implementing Life Recorded in cancer hospitals has been transformative for both patients and healthcare providers. It has reinforced the understanding that healing is a multifaceted process, and true patient-centered care extends beyond medical treatments. The program has not only enriched the lives of those facing terminal illnesses but has also left an indelible mark on the professionals involved, fostering a deeper appreciation for the resilience of the human spirit. As Life Recorded continues to evolve, its integration into mainstream palliative care practices holds the potential to reshape the narrative of end-of-life care. Future advancements may include the incorporation of virtual reality experiences, expanding the program's reach to remote patients, and collaborations with artists and storytellers to enhance the creative elements of the recordings.

As we reflect on the impact of Life Recorded, it becomes a call to action for healthcare systems, policymakers, and society at large. The program challenges us to reevaluate our approach to end-of-life care, urging us to prioritize the preservation of human stories alongside medical interventions. By embracing the principles of Life Recorded, we can collectively strive to create a healthcare landscape that honors the inherent dignity of every individual, even in the face of life's most challenging moments. Life Recorded stands as a beacon of hope in the field of palliative care, demonstrating that the power of storytelling can transform the experience of facing terminal illnesses. As the program continues to evolve, its ripple effect extends beyond hospital walls, inspiring a paradigm shift in the way we approach and understand the end of life. Through the tapestry of audio, video, art, and writing, Life Recorded immortalizes the human spirit, leaving behind a legacy that transcends the confines of mortality.

Life Recorded stands as a testament to the transformative power of human connection and storytelling in the realm of healthcare. In the context of cancer hospitals, where the fragility of life meets the resilience of the human spirit, this program redefines the boundaries of palliative care. Through its innovative multimodal methods, Life Recorded captures not only the medical journey but also the essence of the lives it touches, leaving behind a legacy that transcends the confines of illness and mortality. As Life Recorded continues to unfold, it leaves behind a legacy of compassion, empathy, and transformative care. The program challenges societal taboos surrounding death and invites a collective reflection on the value of preserving human stories. By embracing the principles of Life Recorded, we embark on a journey toward a more compassionate and patient-centered approach to end-of-life care, where the narratives of individuals are not only acknowledged but cherished as enduring testaments to the human spirit.

APPENDIX A

SPIRITUAL CARE ASSESSMENT

SIMPLE ASSESSMENT: FORMAT

Name: ....Floor / Bed Sex Age

Hospital Name
Religious Creed / Philosophy
New / Readmission Date
Relationship to God / Wing / Nature:

SPIRITUALITY
Supreme Authority: Rites
Death Concept:

INFORMATION
Specification of your belief: Special Request
No visit
Source of help: Social assistance

Religious community:
Relationship with the medical / palliative team

MEDICAL
Diagnosis: Level Designated Representative

Palliative Patient (NA / POS / Pre-S)
Medical Situation: Medications (EOL) Advance Directives:

PASTORAL
Value of your religious / philosophical community
Pain
Restrictions
Visits
Confession:

Spiritual Experience: Request:

LET IT GO:
Conduct: Spiritual exercise:

EDUCATION:
Resources: Demography:
Intellectual Guide Pastoral Information
Expressions Mental health

Ecclesiastical / Philosophical Experience

APPENDIX B

CONTRACT LETTERS

Northeastern Conference of Seventh-day Adventists

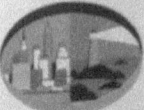

155-50 Merrick Boulevard
Jamaica, N.Y. 11434-5806
Telephone (718) 291-8006

April 29, 1997

TO WHOM IT MAY CONCERN:

We are a tax exempt church under IRC 501 (c), through the General Conference of Seventh-Day Adventist Church, copy of tax exemption certificate is enclosed.

Due to the circumstances of our expanding congregation and services, we have been in need of an additional Minister to attend to the duties and responsibilities of our church functions and expanded membership.

Pastor Reninger Flores is currently attending our Congregation with all religious services as well as funerals, communions and baptisms services; dedication of children to God, preach and teach the Word of God and other duties required from an Ordained Minister.

The duties for which Pastor Flores will be responsible will be carried out by him during 40 hours a week, full time job. With the hours of 9:00 a.m. to 5:00 p.m., the nature of the position will require that he be available for overtime work when needed. Our church is offering this position with a salary of $███████ month. Rev. Flores will not rely on any other income for his support.

My position in the church is Ordained Minister of Religion, a position held since 1975, and also I hold the position of Hispanic Coordinator since 1984 to present.

Sincerely,

urenio Martinez
COORDINATOR/MINISTER

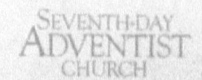

SEVENTH-DAY
ADVENTIST
CHURCH

New York Conference

4930 West Seneca Turnpike
Syracuse, New York 13215-4203
Telephone (315) 469-6921
Fax (315) 469-6724

TO WHOM IT MAY CONCERN:

Please be advised that Mr. Reninger Flores is actively involved in the gospel ministry in behalf of the New York Conference of Seventh-day Adventists. He has been assigned to assist with the ministry of the Buffalo Hispanic Seventh-day Adventist Church located at 1378 South Park Avenue, Buffalo, New York, 14420. Please extend to Mr. Flores every courtesy that his position calls for.

Thanking you for this consideration, I remain,

Sincerely,

Richard

Richard H. Coston, D. Min.
Secretary, New York Conference
of Seventh-day Adventists

APPENDIX C

VERBATIMS

VERBATIM

CHAPLAIN: .... CLIENT'S INITIAL: MG
AGE: ... DATE OF VISIT: 9/25/... MINISTRY SITE: Nazareth
Nursing Home DIAGNOSIS: Unspecified Transient Cerebral Ischemia
DATE SUBMITTED: ... SEX: ... DATE OF ADMISSION: 08/17/...
VERBATIM # 01 MARITAL STATUS: ... DENOMINATION: Catholic

1: **PURPOSE**

2: **BACKGROUND OF PATIENT:** She is a patient located at
the room # ...close to the door and according to the Chart she was
admitted to the Nursing Home on august .... She was born in ...
and her address house is located at..., New York. According to the
documentation she is .. and profess a Catholic religion. When she
admitted to Nazareth Nursing Home, the primary diagnosis is:
Unspecified Transient Cerebral Ischemia, but before she was also
diagnosed with Diabetes mellitus, Senile Dementia Uncomplicated,
Chronic Kidney decease stage II and also during the las two years
she got 6 strokes and the last one happened one week ago that
provoked the total left side paralyzed body.

3. **CONTEXT:** When I came in to the room ... I sow an elderly
lady laid down in her bed with head a little upholding. The room
was co-parted with another resident and looked not very adorned.
on the wall was a small bulletin board without nothing in there,
usually others residents have at least the daily activities schedule, no
flowers on her night table no television and she was barely covered
with a blanket. One lady was sitting down together with her and she
was having a conversation because the lady was able to interact with
me I established a dialog with her, she was very friendly and open to
share their felling and expectations in behalf of the resident whom
was looking me for a while trying to broke a smile and giving me a
welcome to her room. None of the staff was around the patient and
the environment was ready to a conversation.

4. THE INTERACTION

P: Patient

D: Daughter

C: Chaplain

C: (Knocked the open door tree times and came in) Hello, good evening miss Miriam? (Looking at the resident who was laid down her bed) How are you today?

P: (With a Little smile she answered me)! Fine! (Not really audible sound voice)

C. My name is Chaplain Reninger(then I turned my greetings to the lady that was sitting down at the south part of the bed) Hello, How are you?.

D. Pretty good, how are you? (She show me a great smile looking directly my eyes)

C. I am the Chaplain intern in the Nursing Home and I am working together with sister ...She is now on vacation and I am trying to do some kind of job that she usually do, and are. You member of the family of Misses.....

D. Yes, I am her Daughter (addressing with her eyes to the patient), Nice to meet you.

C. Nice to meet you too. (I extended my hand in sign of introducing, and she answered the same way, she was sitting down)

P. (addressing to her daughter)! You are my mom! (At the same time she extend her hand to reach her)

D. No. I am your daughter, I am your daughter (she takes the patient's hand.)

C. How is your mom feeling?

D. She is pretty good

C. Do you think your mother is improving?

D. Yes, definitely, yes. She got 6 strokes and the last one was just last week and affected the left side of her body.

P. (lift up her right hand) you are my mother...

D. Mom. I am not your mother, I am your daughter, OK.

C. Are you the only daughter?

D. Yes, I am, but I have my brother too. He is living in ..., he just left one week ago the day when my mother got the last stroke. C. What is your occupation?

D. I am retired six years ago.

C. Retired from what?

D. National Fuel Company.

C. So. You have time to see your mom very often, aren't?

D. Yes, although I have lot of work to do in my house, and also I have to do extra work in my mother's house, but I take my time to see my mom every day at this place.

C. I really appreciate that concern.

P. (she was moving, showing some kind of uncomfortably whit a blanket and requesting with understandable words and signs, does she wanted to be uncovered.)

D. do you feel too warm. Do you want to get out the blanket?

P. Yes, please.

D. (she took out the blanket) OK. I will fit your blouse so you don't feel cold. OK.

C. What religion does she profess?

D. We are Methodists. She was very active member at my Church. I am attending church every Sunday

C. Is your pastor visiting mom?

D. No he doesn't, I think he is really busy.

C. Well this is my work. I will be visiting your mom, as I can. If you need some prayer, some kind of encouragement for your mom I will be ready. Nice to meet you and God bless you and your mother. See you later.

VERBATIM

Chaplain: .... Client initial: M age: ...Date of visit:
1/23/ Ministry site: Catholic Charities and Refugee Assistance
Program Presenting concern: Date submitted: 1/25/
sex: Male length of stay: 25 minutes Verbatim # 02
Marital status: ... Denomination: Protestant

1. Purpose

This interview has a purpose to show me the level of confidentiality did I get when I spoke with "... How did he respond my interest in being a channel to flow his worries, expectations in personal level and family level? Every suggestions to better response to my client are welcome.

2. Background of client:

My interview with Mathew was in the casual way, I meet him walking in the hallway of the Refugee Center and I had no previous of personal or family information.

3. Context:

It was a round 11:30 am. When I got a break from the Immigration Office at Catholic charities located at cross the door. I crossed the main door at the Center I started greeting in the hallway all students that I meet them in my previous visit to the classrooms. After a while I saw a white guy standing up together a cylindrical container with full of cloths and some breads on the cover I guess with the intention to pick up something from the container. He was watching me too. He was wearing a black jacket and his smiling face gave a good opportunity to go close to him and introduce myself.

4. Interaction:

C: Chaplain E. Student
C1 Hello, my name is Chaplain Reninger (walking closer toward him)
E1
C2
E2
C3
High level, aren't? And you are speaking good and understandable English, believe me.
Hello, I am M.., nice to meet you
Nice to meet you too. Are a student in the Center?
Yes, I am. I am waiting Teacher A... to go back to my class. Oh, I know you are in the 3rd level of English I mean the

E3 Thanks. I'm preparing to the test to be an American Citizen, and Teacher A... is graciously giving me the clue to respond all the questions in order to pass the test.

C4.
E4
C5
remember but I am pretty sure you will succeed in your test. What about your family?
Do you have already the date of your test.
Not yet, but I want to be ready when it comes to me..
I know are around 100 questions and they are not easy to

E5 I Have 11 kids. Two of them are in College. Buffalo Sate College, The rest are in high school and middle School others are still little ones. My wife in taking care of the little ones in my home. C6 I see. E6 I just moved to my new apartment. Before I was living in Amherst, but recently I got another apartment in Tonawanda where

I just moved and is more easier for me to came to the Center when I have my English class. I like Buffalo.

C7. You said you like Buffalo.

E7 Yes, Buffalo reminds me my old country. I am from Byelorussia. When do we have snowy time in Byelorussia is the same here, and I know because I talk by phone with my relatives many times during the month.. But in the future I would like to move to North Carolina because I have lot of friends from my same country living there. Also the same religion.

C8 What religion do you practice?

E8 I am protestant

C9 Protestant, what kind of protestant. Evangelical, Pentecostal, Methodist, Baptist..?

E9 No. I really don't know what kind of church I am going. (He looked a little confuse) is located very close to Elmwood Avenue. What about you, are you Catholic?

C10

E10

C11

E11

Yes, 50 kilometers from my town there is a big Adventist Church with lot of people also I have a friend who is assisting to this church. I never went to this church. (Pause), but I know about your church. And where you came from?

C12 I am from Peru, in South America.

E12 Peru, is close to Argentina, Brazil .....(Pause) I love the way you guys play soccer. I love Peruvian soccer. In my country usually I played soccer but here is not very common.

C13 Ok. M..., it was a pleasure to talk with you. My best wishes in your next citizenship test. I have to go back to the Immigration office to continue my work. We had an interesting conversation. E13 Thanks for talking to me (smiling)

C14 By, By.

5. Assessment of client / Situation

M...was worried about his preparation to the citizenship test. As a responsible student he was waiting to go back to class after the brake. Also he looks very confident about the course of the family.
I am member of the Adventist Church You mean SDA Church.
Yes, do you know this church, did you hear before?
Yes I did. In B.. near to my town. Let me think...Let me think.
Explaining his great accomplishment in reference to his kids." All of them in school" sounds from him a successful expression. The geographic location of Buffalo is for him a strategic place to prosper but he misses his friends that are now living at ..

6. Spiritual Assessment

I found in him a hard desire to succeed. His great will to learn English, his indubitable desire to pass the upcoming test for him to become an American citizen and all kids in school shows for me he is going forward and he will be a successful citizen and a strong family in the society.

7. Theological Reflection

Mathew for me is the typical immigrant that is ready to make changes in America. He is a believer and to be successful immigrant we need strong faith in God first of all and then in oneself. He has in his hands all this tools. God is blessing me with this encounter because I learned from this stranger man his openness braking his private life in my hands and give me the great meaningful opportunity to push him a little bit more on n the road of the success not just for him if not for the entire family. I think the gift of hearing from the strange voice is the gift from heaven to live in this world where the privacy covers the life of the dying society where public realm is shadowed.

8. Identity of the Chaplain

All my conversation I tried to encourage him to go ahead in his purpose to learn, to succeed, and to be involved in the American life. And also I tried to show him that nothing is easy especially when you are trying to get a real purpose in life. The obstacles are normal in life but need to overcome for own good. I learned that in the constantly world of complaints there people smiling, with strong faith, and good desire of prosperity... My question is why another people see the obstacles as a problem? Do I in my life looking in the same way?

9. Follow Up

I am not sure I will see again this client but in my next interview I would to enter more in his spiritual; background and see the secret of his strength.

10. Recording the Visit

No record was kept from this visit.

REFERENCE LIST

REFERENCE LIST

Abelmann, N.; Davis, S.; Finnegan, C.; Miller, P. (1 June 2009). What is StoryCorps,

Anyway? *Oral History Review.* 36(2): 255–260.

ACA, (2014). ACA code of ethics as approved by the ACA governing council. Retrieved from https://www.counseling. org/docs/default-source/ethics/2014-aca-code-of-ethics. pdf?sfvrsn=fde89426 5

Adnoy, E, K., Sundfor, B., Karlsson, B., Raholm, M, B., & Arman, M. (2012). Recognition as a valued human being: perspectives of mental health services users. Nursing Ethics, 19(3), 357-368.

Adshead, G. (2012). Studying the mind: Ethical issues and guidance in mental health research. Clinical Ethics, 3(3), 141-144.

Alfieri, D.L. (2015). Marketing plan research and assessment (Definition of quantitative research). Retrieved from https://www. sciencedirect.com/topics/social-sciences/ quantitative-research.

Alliedhealth. (2019, August 4). Healthcare in the age of data. How to complywiththeHIPAAsecurityrule.Retrievedfromhttps://www. insureon.com/blog/how-to-comply-with-hipaa-security-rule

Anandarajah, G., & Hight, E. (2001). Spirituality and medical practice: Using the HOPE questions as a practical tool for spiritual assessment. Retrieved from https://www.aafp.org/afp

Asato, Jon. (2019). Here I am the lord: An invitation to become a prayer chaplain. Retrieved from https//.www.unityoffairfax.org

Asco. (2020). How cancer affects family life. American Society of Clinical Oncology. Retrieved from https://www.cancer.net/coping-with-cancer

Association of Professional Chaplains. (2020). The meaning and practice of spiritual care [White paper]. Retrieved from https:// www.professionalchaplains.org/files/ resources/program development/starting chaplaincy program/white paper text only. pdf.page 7

Bauer, A. (2014). Spotlight: Oncology social worker part 1, A Q&A. Retrieved from https://www.cancer.net

Beauchamp, L. T., & Childress J. F. (2012). Methods and principle of biomedical ethics (7th ed.). Oxford, England: Oxford University Press.

Bibleref(2020). Got questions Ministries. Retrieved from https:// www.bibleref.com/2-Corinthians/13/2-Corinthians-13-5.html. Paragraph 2

Borneman, T. (2018). Assessment of spirituality in older adults: FICA spiritual history tool. Retrieved from https://consultgeri. org/try-this/specialty-practice

Brannan, S., Campbell, R., Davies, M., English, V., Mussell, R., & Sheather, J. (2016, June). BMA end-of–life care and physician-assisted dying project.Journal of Medical Ethics, 42(6), 409–10. doi:10.1136/medethics-2016-103608

Brennan, M. (2014). The A–Z of death and dying: Social, medical, and cultural aspects. Santa Barbara, CA: ABC-CLIO/Greenwood.

Brown, C. G. (2013). The healing gods: Complementary and alternative medicine in Christian America. New York, NY: Oxford University Press. Retrieved from https://www.nccih. nih.gov/research.3/29/2020

Bultz, D. B. (2016). Cancer care and the role of psychosocial oncology: Where are we and where are we going. Asia-Pacific Journal of Oncology Nursing, 3(2), 118-120.

Buse, N. A., Burker, E. J., & Bernacchio, C. (2013, April). Cultural variation in resilience as a response to traumatic experience. The

Journal of Rehabilitation, 79(2), 15–23. Retrieved from www.questia,com

Bussinessjargon(2020). Liker scale level of measurement. Retrieved from https://businessjargons.com/likert-scale, paragraph 1, 7/22/2020

Cadge, W. (2012). Paging God: Religion in the halls of medicine. Chicago, IL: University of Chicago Press.

Carlick, A. & Biley, F. C. (2004). Thoughts on the therapeutic use of narrative in the promotion of coping in cancer care. *European Journal of Cancer Care.* 13 (4): 308-317.

Cemental, R. (2019). The psychological effects of a hospital stay on seniors [Weblog]. Retrieved from https://www.caringseniorservice.com/blog/the-psychological-effect-of-a-hospital-stay-on-seniors

Chelf, J. H.; Deshler, A.; Hillman, S.; Durazo-Arvizu, R. (2000). Storytelling. *Cancer Nursing.* (23)1: 1-5.

Christianity (2020).Matthew Henry's Bible Commentary (concise). Commentary on Mark 4:1-20. Paragraph 1. Retrieved from https://www.christianity.com/bible/commentary.

Chowdhury, A. R. (2016, December 23). Purify your mind soul with these 4 techniques [Webpage]. Onlymyhealth. Retrieved from https://www.onlymyhealth.com/ purify-your-mind-and-soul-with-4-techniques-1482474401

Crogan, N. L.; Evans, B. C.; Bendel, R. (2008). Storytelling Intervention for Patients with Cancer. *Oncology Nursing Forum.* 35(2): 265-272.

DeFranzo.E.S. (2011). What's the difference between qualitative and quantitative research? Retrieved from www.snapsurveys.com

Delgado-Guay, M. O., Parsons, H, A., Hui, D., De la Cruz, M. G., Thorney, S., & Bruera, E. (2013, August 1). Spirituality, religiosity, and spiritual pain among caregivers of patients with advanced cancer. American Journal of Hospice & Palliative Medicine, 30(5), 455-461. Retrieved from https://journals.sagepub.com/doi/ 10.1177/1049909112458030

DeMarinis, V. (2018). Mental health diagnosis: Is it relative or universal in relation to culture? In M. Stenmark, S. Fuller, & U. Zackariasson (Eds.) Relativism and post-truth in contemporary society (pp. 101-121). Cham, Switzerland: Palgrave Macmillan. Retrieved from https://link.springer.com/ chapter/10.1007/978-3-319-96559-8 7

Donn, L., & Martin, P. (2020). The legend of the Trojan war for kids: Greek mythology for kids and teachers. Retrieved from http:// paigeentwistle.com/greek-myths/the-tojan-war.

Dörnbrak, M. (2020). Module 4/lesson 2: The 7 principles of discipleship (pp. 17-18: Acts of the Apostles). Retrieved from http://www.discipleshipcourse.org/images/ pdf/modul04/02-The 7 Principles of Discipleship.pdf

Downing, J., Marston, J., Muckaden, M. A., Boucher, S., Cardoz, M., Nkosi, B., . . . Tilve, P. (2014, March 31). Transforming children's palliative care-from ideas to action: Highlights from the first ICPCN conference on children's palliative care. Ecancermedicalscience, 8, 415. National Center for Biotechnology Information, Bethesda MD. Retrieved from www.ncbi.nlm.nih. gov/pmc/articles/PMC3971869/

Duru, A. (2016, November-December). Spiritual care and metal health: What the research tell us [Webpage]. Mental Health: Issues and Opportunities. The National Association of Catholic Chaplains. Retrieved from https://www.nacc.org/vision/november-december-2016/ spiritual-care-mental-health-research-tells-us/

Edmonds, M. (2011). A theological diagnosis: A new direction on genetic therapy, 'disability' and the ethics of healing. London: England: Jessica Kingsley.

Edwards, A., Pang, N., Shiu, V., & Chan, C. (2010, December). The understanding and the potential role of spiritual care in end-of-life and palliative care: A meta-study of quality research. Palliative Medicine, 24(8), 753-770. Retrieved from https:// pubmed.ncbi.nlm.nih.gov/20659977/

Eilberg, A. (2000). When someone you love is dying [Booklet]. Woodstock, VT: Jewish Lights.

Ellison, L., Gask, L., Bakerly, N, D., & Roberts, J. (2012, December). Meeting the mental needs of people with chronic obstructive pulmonary disease: A qualitative study. Chronic Illness, 8(4), 308–20. Retrieved from https://pubmed.ncbi.nlm. nih.gov/22659349/

Fairman, N., & Irwin, S. A. (2014, March 24). Attending to the mental suffering of patients with progressive medical illness. Psychiatric Times, 31(3), 1-6.

Ferrell, B, R.,Coyle, N. (2006). Textbook of palliative nursing. Oxford. Principles of patient and family assessment. University Press Inc. page 58, 59

Frankl, Viktor E. (1962). Man's Search for Meaning: an Introduction to Logotherapy. Boston: Beacon Press.

Freund, A. (2015). Under Storytelling's Spell? Oral History in a Neoliberal Age. *Oral History Review.* 42(1): 96–132.

Gaithri, A, F. (2012). The roads less traveled: Mapping some pathways on the global mental health research roadmap. Transcultural Psychiatry, 49(3-4), 396-417. Retrieved from https://journals. sagepub.com

Ghasemian, K.; Estahbanati, M. A. E. (2019). The Effectiveness of Storytelling on Reducing Depression in Cancer Patients. *Humanities and Innovation.* 6(9): 278-284.

Ghoshal, S., Miriyala, R., Elangovan, A., & Rai, B. (2016, July-Sept). Why newly diagnosed cancer patients require supportive care? An audit from a regional cancer center in India. Indian Journal of Palliative Care, 22(3), 326–330. Retrieved from https://www. ncbi.nlm.nih.gov/pmc/articles/PMC4973495/

Glickman, M. S. (2012, March 23). We know death is coming—for all of us—so why does it make us so sad when somebody dies? The Seattle Times. Retrieved from https://www.seattletimes. com/seattle-news/why-does-death-make-us-so-sad/

Gómez, S. (2019, December 23). Hanukkah meaning of each candle, traditions, and how is celebrated. Latin Times. Retrived from https://www.latintimes.com /hanukkah-meaning-each-candle-traditions-and-how-its-celebrated-429085

Gould, N., Huxley P., & Tew, J. (2007). Finding a direction for social research in mental health: Establishing priorities and developing capacity. Journal of Social Work, 7(2), 179-196.

Gramling, D., & Gramling, R. (2019). Palliative Care Conversations: Clinical and applied linguistic perspectives. Boston, MA: Mouton De Gruyter. Retrieved from https://www.amazon.com/Palliative-Care-Conversations-Linguistic-Perspectives/dp/1501512684

Groth-Marnat, G. (2009). The Handbook of psychological assessment (5th ed.).Hoboken, NJ: Wiley. Retrieved from http://www. dilayeldogan.com/wp-content/uploads. 4 /21/2020

Gunten, C. F. von. (2020). National consensus project definition of palliative care. Stanford School of Medicine. Retrieved from https://palliative.stanford.edu/ overview-of-palliative-care/national-consensus-project-definition-of-palliative-care/ Halamish, L, D., & Hermoni, D. (2007). The weeping willow: Encounters with grief. Oxford, Egland: Oxford University Press. Harris, D, M. (2008). Contemporary issues in health care law and ethics (3rd Ed.). Chicago, IL: Health Administration.

Harris, J. I., Erbes, C. R., Engdahl, B. E., Thuras, P., Murray-Swank, N., Grace, D., . . . Le, T. (2011, April). The effectiveness of a trauma focused spiritually integrated intervention for veterans exposed to trauma. Journal of Clinical Psychology, 67(4), 425-38. Retrieved from https://www.ncbi.nlm.nih.gov/pubmed/21294116/

Hodge, D. R. (2006, Oct). A template for spiritual assessment: A review of the JCAHO requirements and guidelines for implementations. Social Work, 51(4), 317-26. Retrieved from https://pubmed.ncbi.nlm.nih.gov/17152630/

Hurley, J., Linsley, P., & Macleod, S. (2012). The movement of knowledge and benefit: the product of applied ethics and emotional intelligence to mental health research. Journal of Research in Nursing, 17(5), 455-463.

Ingvarsdotter, K., Johnsdotter, S., & Ostman, M. (2012, January). Lost in interpretation: The use of interpreters in research on mental ill health. International Journal of Social Psychiatry, 58(1), 34-40.

Isay, D. (2016). *Callings: The Purpose and Passion of Work.* Penguin Press.

Issues in palliative care communication, transition, and end-of-life medical care. (2013). Strategies and goals of palliative care section, paragraph 2. Retrieved from https://s3.amazonaws.com/ EliteCME WebSite 2013/f/pdf/NSC07PCI12.pdf

Johns, C. (2004). Being Mindful, Easing Suffering: Reflections on palliative care. London, England: Kingley. Retrived from https://www.worldcat.org/title/being-mindful-easing-suffering-reflections-on-palliative-care

Kajiwara, K., Kako, J., Miyashita, M. (2019, July 18). Response to: "Caring for the person with cancer and the role of digital technology in supporting carers.". Supportive Care in Cancer, 28 (3), 961.

Kaslow, N. J. (2014, April). Our opportunity to reduce suicide. Monitor on Psychology, 45(4), 5. Washington DC.

Kidder, S. J. (2015, March). Planning a sermonic year. Ministry Magazine. International journal for pastors.

Kirsch, A. (2012, November 6). Standing on one foot. Tablet Magazine. Retrieved from https://www.tabletmag.com/ jewish-life-and-religion.

Kitchener, C. (2018, January). Spiritual but not religious. The Atlantic. Retrieved from: https://www.theatlantic.com/ membership/archive/2018/01/what-it-means-to-be-spiritual-but-not-religious. Koenig, H. (2011). Spirituality and health research: Methods, measurements, statistics and resources. West Conshohocken, PA: Templeton Foundation Press.

Kostelnik, M., J., Soderman, A. K., Whiren, A. P., & Rupiper, M. L. (2018). Guiding children's social development & learning: Theory and skills. Boston, MA: Cengage Learning.

Kunner, S. (1999). Speak the language of healing: Living with breast cancer without going to war. Berkeley, CA: Conari Press. Retrieved from https://www.goodreads.com/book/show

Laing, C. M.; Moules, N. J.; Sinclair, S.; Estefan, A. (2019). Digital Storytelling as a Psychosocial Tool for Adult Cancer Survivors. *Oncology Nursing Forum.* 46(2): 147-154.

Larimore, W. (2017, May 10). Spiritual assessment in clinical practice: An evidence based approach [Webpage]. Medical Missions. LaRocca-Pitts, M. A. (2009). FACT: Taking a spiritual history in a clinical setting. Journal of health care chaplaincy, 15(1), 1–12. Retrieved from https://www.tandfonline.com/doi/abs/10.1080/08854720802698350?mobileUi=0&journalCode=whcc20 Lenegan, B. (2018, May 4). Interview by R. Flores. Spiritual Care Assessment. Roswell Main Hospital.

Lenegan, B., & Clearence, D. (2015). Caring across cultures and belief systems: Buddhism Roswell Park Cancer Institute, Department of Diversity.

Levy, D. (2011, Nov 29). Patients desire prayer in the hospital [Webpage]. Retrieved from https://www.drdlevy.com/?s=Patient+desire+prayer+in+the+hospital

Lith, V, T. (2014). A meeting with I-thou: Exploring the intersection between mental health recovery and art making through a co- operative inquiry. Advancement of Mental Health, 4(3), 179-182.

LosCalzo, M. J. (2008). Hematology am soc hemato: Palliative care an historical perspective. Retrieved from Hospicebuffalo.com/patients-and-caregivers

Macauley, R. C. (2018). Ethics in palliative care: A complete guide. Oxford, England: Oxford University Press.

MacKinlay, E. B., & Trevitt, C. (2007). Spiritual care and aging in a secular society. Medical Journal of Australia, 186(10), S74.

Mandal, J., Ponnambath, D, K., & Parija, S. C. (2016, January-June). Utilitarian and deontological ethics in medicine. Tropical Parasitology, 6(1), 5-7. Retrieved from https://www.ncbi.nlm.nih.gov/pmc/articles/PMC4778182/

Mayavu, M. (2017). Uncommodified blackness: The African male experience in Australia and New Zealand. Cham, Switzerland: Palgrave McMillian.

McSherry, W., Draper, P., & Kendrik, D. (2002). The construct validity of a rating scale designed to assess spirituality and spiritual care. International Journal of Nursing Studies, 39(7), 723-734.

Meador, K, G., & Levin, J, S. (2012). Healing to all their flesh: Jewish and Christian perspectives on spirituality, theology, and health. West Conshohocken, PA: Templeton Press.

Medina, C. (2020). Belief and traditions that impact Latino healthcare. New Orleans, LA: Louisiana State University School of Public Health, Delta Region Aids Education Center. Retrieved from https://www.medschool.lsuhsc.edu/physiology/ docs/Belief%20 and%20Traditions%20that%20impact%20the%20Latino%20 Healthcare.pdf?TB iframe=true&width=370.8&height=658.8

Morris, D. N. (2013, March). Perceptions of the use of spirituality, and spiritual care in occupational therapy practice. 29(1):60-77. Retrieved from https://www.researchgate.net/ publication/280092111 Perceptions of Spirituality and Spiritual Care in Occupational Therapy Practice

Morrison, R. S. (2013). Models of palliative care delivery in the United State. Current Opinion in Supportive and Palliative Care, 7(2), 201-206.

Neukrug,S,E.,Faucett,C.R.(2010)Essentials of Testing and Assessment. A Practical guide for counselors.social workers and psichologists. Brooks/Cole Cengage learning, CA.

Novotney, A. (2014, July-August). Integrated care at work. Monitor on Psychology, 45(7), 46. Retrieved from https://www.apa.org/monitor/2014/07-08/integrated-care

Office of Research Integrity. (2019, April 15). Business and financial issues. Retrieved from http://ori.hhs.gov/education

Onyenali, R. (2013). The trilogy of parables in Mt 21:28-22:14: From a Matthean perspective. Frankfurt am Main, Germany: Peter Lang Press.

Paice,A, J.,Fine,G, P.(2006). Pain at the end of life. Textbook of palliative nursing. Oxford University Press. Page 131

Parker, R. A. (2019). The Universalist pocket guide. Bylaws and rules. Page 4. Unitarian Universalist Association. Boston MA.

Peteet, J. R., & D'Ambra, M. N. (2011). The soul of medicine: Spiritual perspectives and clinical practice. Baltimore, MD: Johns Hopkins University Press.

Piotrowski, L, F. (2017, November-December). The chaplain's role as catalyst for 'good death'. Health Progress: Journal of the Catholic Health Association of the United States. Retrieved from https://www.chausa.org/publications/health-progress/article/november-december-2017/the-chaplain's- role-as-catalyst-for-good-death

Presser, S.,Couper,P.M.,Lessler, T, J.,Martin, E.,Martin J.,Rothgeb,M,J.,Singer, E.(2004). Methods for Testing and Evaluating survey questions. Public Opinion Quarterly, vol 68, Issue 1, page 110

Prusak, J. (2016). Differential diagnosis of "religious or spiritual problem"—Possibilities and limitations implied by the V-code 62.89 in DSM-5. Psychiatria Polska, 50(1), 175–186. Retrieved from www.psychiatriapolska.pl/uploads/images/ PP 1 2016/ ENGver175Prusak PsychiatrPol2016v50i1.pdf

Quill, E. T., & Miller, F. G. (2014). Palliative care and ethics. New York, NY: Oxford University Press.

Rapp-Paglicci, L., Stewart, C., Rowe, W., & Miller, M. J. (2011). Addressing the Hispanic delinquency and mental health relationship through cultural arts programming: A research note from the prodigy evaluation. Journal of Contemporary Criminal Justice, 27(1), 110-121.

Reid, M. (2016). Clinical and social contexts of ethical issues in mental health care. AMA Journal of Ethics, 18(6), 567-571. Rodgers, M. (2013). Spiritual care policy. Aberdeen, Scotland: Aberdeen Royal Infirmary.

Rugkasa, J., & Canvin, K. (2011). Research mental health in minority ethnic communities:

Reflections on recruitment. Qualitative Health Research, 21(1), 132-143.

Ryu, S.; Price, S. K. (2021). Embodied storytelling and meaning-making at the end of life: VoicingHan avatar life-Review for palliative care in cancer patients. *Arts Health*. 23: 1-15.

Schantz, B. (2015, July-September) Sabbath School Bible Study Guide: Biblical Missionaries. Retrieved from https://www. ssnet. org/study-guides/lesson-archives/2010-2019/2015- q3-biblical-missionaries/

Schulenberg, S. E., Baczwaski, J. B., & Buchanan, M. E. (2013, May 25). Measuring search for meaning: A factor-analytic evaluation of the Seeking of Noetic Goals Test (SONG). Journal of Happiness Studies, 15, 693–715. Retrieved from https://www. researchgate.net/publication

Schultz, M., Lulav-Grinwald, D., & Bar-Sela, G. (2014, April 8). Cultural differences in spiritual care: Findings on an Israeli oncologic questionnaire examining patient interest in spiritual care. BMC Palliative Care, 13(1), 19. Retrieved from https:// www.ncbi.nlm.nih.gov/pmc/articles/PMC4108186/

Seguin,M.(1992). A Gentle death. Patient and doctors. Page 34 paragraph,1.

Sharma, H., Varma, J., Anusha, P., & Bharti, S. (2013, January). End of life care: Indian perspective. Indian Journal of Psychiatry, 55(6), 293-98. doi:10.4103/0019-5545.105554

Shiel, W. C., Jr. (2018). Medical definition of psycho-oncology. Midterms medical dictionary a-z list. Retrieved from https://www.medicinenet.com/script// main/art.asp?articlekey=33446

Simcha, P. R. (2019). Jewish views of the afterlife (3rd ed.). Lanham:MD: Rowman & Littlefield.

Siouta, N., Van Beek, K., van der Eerden, M. E., Preston, N., Hasselaar, J. G., Hughes, S., . . . Menten, J. (2016, July 8). Integrated Palliative Care in Europe: A qualitative Systematic literature review of empirically tested models in cancer and chronic disease. BMC Palliative Care 15(56). Retrieved from https:// bmcpalliatcare.biomedcentral.com/articles/10.1186/ s12904-016-0130-7

Stanford University. (2019, April 15). What are the basic principles of medical ethics? Retrieved from http://web.stanford.edu

Stark, C. A., & Bonner, D. C. (2010). Handbook of spirituality: Belief systems, societal impact and roles in coping. New York, NY: Nova Science.

Stoltzfus, M. (2013). Chronic illness, spirituality, and healing: Diverse disciplinary, religious and cultural perspectives. New York, NY: Palgrave Macmillan., pages 119-216

Taylor, J, S. (2013). The metaphysics and ethics of death. New York, NY: Oxford University Press.

Underwood, L. G. (1999). A working model of health: Spirituality and religiousness as resources: Applications to persons with disability. Journal of Religion Disability & Health, 3(3). Retrieved from https://www.researchgate.net/publication/252237323 A Working Model of Health Spirituality and Religiousness as Resources Applications to Persons with Disability United States Conference of Catholic Bishops. (2009). Ethical and religious directives for catholic health care services (5th ed.). Washington DC: Author. Retrieved from www. usccbpublishing.org

United States Senate. (2020). Office of the Senate Chaplain. Retrieved from https://www.senate.gov/reference/office/chaplain.htm U.S. Department of Health and Human Services, Office of Disease

Prevention and Health Promotion. (2019, April 15). The Joint commission. Retrieved from http:// healthfinder.gov

Village, A., & Piedmont, R. (Eds.). (2013). Research in the social scientific study of religion (Vol. 24). Leiden, Netherlands: Brill. Watson, M. (2019, July 22). About this journal [Abstract]. Psycho- Oncology. Retrieved from https://onlinelibrary.wiley. com/journal/10991611

White, E. G. (1892). Gospel workers 1892. Battle Creek, MI: Review & Herald.

White, E. G. (1911). The acts of the apostles. Mountain View, CA: Pacific Press.

White, E. G. (1923). Counsels on health. Mountain View, CA: Pacific Press.

White, E. G. (1930). Messages to young people. Hagerstown, MD: Review & Herald.

White, E. G. (1946). Evangelism. Washington, DC: Review & Herald.

White, E. G. (1988). Lift Him up. (Hagerstown, MD: Review & Herald.

Wilson-Stronks, A., Schyve, P., Cordero, C. L., Rodríguez, I., & Youdelman, M. (2010). Advancing effective communication, cultural competence, and patient-and family-centered care: A roadmap for hospitals. Oakbrook Terrace, IL: The Joint Commission.

Woodley, M. (2011) The Gospel of Mathew: God with us. Downers Grove, IL: InterVarsity Press.

World Health Organization (2021). Quality Of Life: Measuring Quality of Life. https://www.who.int/tools/whoqol